Partial Dentures

Partial Dentures

D. J. NEILL DFC MDS FDSRCS
Professor of Prosthetic Dentistry
University of London
Head of Department of Prosthetic Dentistry
Guy's Hospital, London

J. D. WALTER DDS FDSRCSE
Senior Lecturer
Department of Prosthetic Dentistry
Guy's Hospital, London

SECOND EDITION

Blackwell Scientific Publications
Oxford London Edinburgh
Boston Melbourne

© 1977, 1983 Blackwell Scientific
Publications
Editorial offices:
Osney Mead, Oxford OX2 0EL
8 John Street, London WC1N 2ES
9 Forrest Road, Edinburgh EH1 2QH
52 Beacon Street, Boston
  Massachusetts 02108, USA
99 Barry Street, Carlton
  Victoria 3053, Australia

All rights reserved. No part of this
publication may be reproduced, stored
in a retrieval system, or transmitted, in
any form or by any means, electronic,
mechanical, photocopying, recording or
otherwise without the prior permission
of the copyright owner.

First published 1977
Second edition 1983

Printed and bound in Great Britain at
the Alden Press, Oxford

DISTRIBUTORS

USA
  Blackwell Mosby Book Distributors
  11830 Westline Industrial Drive
  St Louis, Missouri 63141

Canada
  Blackwell Mosby Book Distributors
  120 Melford Drive, Scarborough
  Ontario, M1B 2X4

Australia
  Blackwell Scientific Book
    Distributors
  31 Advantage Road, Highett
  Victoria 3190

British Library
Cataloguing in Publication Data

Neill, D. J.
  Partial dentures.— 2nd ed.
  1. Partial dentures—
    Laboratory manuals
  I. Title   II. Walter, J. D.
  617.6′92   RK656

ISBN 0–632–01025–8

Contents

Preface — vii

Introduction — 1

Clinical stage 1 — 5
History, examination and treatment planning. Primary impressions. Face bow record. Jaw relationships.

Clinical stage 1(a) — 20
Registering centric jaw relationship.

Laboratory procedures 1 — 23
Casting the impressions. Preparation of occlusion rims. Surveying the casts. Mounting study casts.

Partial denture design — 30
Classification of the partially edentulous mouth. Outline saddle areas and plan support. Select path of insertion and survey cast. Providing resistance to displacement away from supporting tissues. Direct retainers. Indirect retainers. Providing resistance to movement in the horizontal plane. Clasp design. The design of connectors. Construction of special trays.

Clinical stage 2 — 49
Mouth preparation for partial dentures. General care. Specific preparation. Preparation of occlusal table. Modification of occlusal form. Modification of proximal and buccolabial form. Obtaining working impressions.

Laboratory procedures 2 — 57
Preparation of master casts. Surveying casts and outline design. Modifying the master casts. Preparing the investment cast. Preparing wax pattern. Spruing. Investing and casting the metal framework. Finishing the framework for insertion in the mouth.

Clinical stage 3 — 72
Trial insertion of the cast framework. Special problems of the distal extension saddle

Laboratory procedures 3(a) — 79
Adding acrylic tray to the distal extension framework.

Clinical stage 3(a) — 80
Description of the fluid wax technique for recording an impression of distal extension saddle areas.

v

Contents

Laboratory procedures 3(b) — 83
Altering the cast by means of the fluid wax impression.

Clinical stage 4 — 84
Jaw relationships. Selection of teeth.

Laboratory procedures 4 — 86
Setting the teeth for trial insertion.

Clinical stage 5 — 87
Trial insertion.

Laboratory procedures 5 — 88
Processing the denture.

Clinical stage 6 — 90
Fitting the completed dentures. Denture and oral hygiene. Instructions concerning the use of the dentures.

Clinical stage 7 — 94
Adjustment of the denture.

Appendix — 97
Acrylic partial dentures.

Special notes on specific forms of partial denture design — 104
Two part dentures. Hinged flange dentures. The Swinglock Denture. Disjunct dentures.

References and further reading — 115

Index — 117

Preface

There are many admirable textbooks concerned with the restoration of the partially edentulous mouth but few which seek to set down in a succinct fashion the objectives of each clinical stage followed by an illustrated narrative of the clinical and laboratory stages of partial denture construction. We have attempted to fill this gap in prosthetic literature and hope that we may have dispelled some of the mysticism which so often surrounds this subject. Despite the enormous variety of permutations of edentulous spaces (Cummer has calculated the possible number at 131 068), of tooth alignment and occlusal relationships, the restoration of the partially edentulous mouth depends upon the understanding of relatively few fundamental principles which have been enumerated in the text. Although written primarily for undergraduate students, it is hoped that many practitioners will find it a valuable aid to their postgraduate studies.

We are particularly indebted to Mr John Glaysher who, in addition to carrying out most of the technical procedures, has also been responsible for nearly all of the photographs illustrating the text. We are also grateful to the staff of the Department of Dental Photography of Guy's Hospital Dental School for their help. Finally, we wish to express our appreciation to our secretaries for their painstaking preparation of the manuscript and to our wives for typing and proof reading.

London 1983 *D.J.Neill*
 J.D.Walter

Introduction

Although the provision of a partial denture may represent the completion of a course of dental treatment, the planning of the prosthetic restoration should commence with the patient's first visit.

We should, at the outset, consider the reasons for replacing teeth by means of a partial denture. Patients commonly seek treatment when an edentulous space is visible or when they have difficulty in eating. There are, however, other indications for treatment which may lead the dentist to prescribe dentures.

If supraeruption, tilting or drifting of teeth is anticipated, a prosthesis may be provided to maintain the integrity of the dental arch.

Where, due to the loss of posterior teeth, abnormal function of the temporomandibular joint may be induced or uneven forces applied to an opposing complete denture, it is important to establish an even occlusion throughout the arch. A prosthesis may be recommended to splint the teeth as part of the treatment of periodontal disease.

Any prosthesis placed in the mouth constitutes a potential hazard to the health of the teeth and their supporting tissues: this can be minimised by careful design of the appliance and instructing the patient in the care of his denture and oral hygiene. The likelihood of the patient heeding this advice must be an important factor in deciding whether or not to proceed with treatment.

Patients must understand the need for their partial dentures and the importance of achieving a high standard of oral hygiene at the outset. The consequences of failing to play their part in maintaining these high standards of oral and denture care should be explained. Plaque should be disclosed and the patient instructed in oral hygiene measures. They must understand the need for the provision of satisfactory dentures and be agreeable to undergo such treatment.

Patients who have neglected their mouths for many decades often show the greatest reluctance to being parted from their remaining teeth. However, unless a sufficient number of teeth suitably positioned in each quadrant can be restored, together with their supporting tissues, the wise prosthetist will decline the provision of partial dentures. Those foolish enough to acquiesce in the provision of partial dentures where the remaining teeth and supporting alveolar bone fall short of the requirements of support and retention, will gradually convert the partial denture into complete dentures. During this period adverse changes will occur so that the contour of the bone around the periodontally-involved last teeth will become excessive. There is also the possibility that periodontal abscesses will add to the patient's discomfort.

There are certain situations which should be avoided:

1 The retention of lower canines and incisors is of questionable value. No undercuts exist for the purpose of denture retention and unless unsightly embrasure hooks or rest seats are prepared they can supply no support. It is well-nigh impossible to provide a partial lower denture with a mucosa support element which maintains satisfactory posterior occlusion over a long period. When the opposing jaw is edentulous the anterior alveolar process is stimulated to resorb and to be replaced by fibrous tissue, hence the flabby ridge. If partial dentures are to be provided under these circumstances, preparation of the teeth to facilitate support and retention is essential and very frequent inspection of the dentures is necessary so that the dentures can be rebased to counter the effect of bone resorption.

2 Retaining isolated teeth in otherwise edentulous mouths is usually contra-indicated. They contribute little or no support or retentive function and have an adverse effect upon the stability of the opposing denture. In addition they tend to stimulate the resorption of the opposing alveolar bone which bears the thrust of the occlusion.

In the above situations consideration may be given to the possibility of utilising the endodontically treated roots of some of the teeth for purposes of support of an overdenture.

Malaligned and overerupted teeth not only prejudice the design of partial dentures, but also interfere with the articulation of the teeth. If they cannot be modified in form they may be better extracted.

With bounded saddles, there may be a choice between fixed and removable prostheses. Bridges have the advantage of minimal bulk and, because of the absence of extracoronal retainers, are usually of superior appearance.

Many patients prefer the sense of permanence which a fixed prosthesis gives. However, the success of bridgework depends upon the abutment teeth having an intact bony support and the patient adopting the most scrupulous standards of oral hygiene. Because a fixed bridge cannot be removed inflammatory changes taking place beneath it cannot be checked and treatment measures instituted.

Partial dentures usually derive their support from a large number of teeth and have the advantage of being braced by components on both sides of the dental arch. Where multiple saddles need to be restored, a partial denture may provide the treatment of choice.

There is, of course, a great deal of satisfaction to be gained from restoring a mouth in the ideal manner. However, the more patients who have elaborate and time-consuming programmes of treatment provided, the fewer of the population will receive care. Because of the limitations in dental manpower and the high cost involved, the treatment prescribed may often have to be a compromise. This, however, should never result in one losing sight of the essential principles of partial denture design which must always be upheld.

Clinical stage 1

HISTORY, EXAMINATION AND TREATMENT PLAN

History

The compilation of a patient's history falls into three well-defined phases:
1. Personal details.
2. Relevant medical history.
3. Dental history.

Personal details

These include name, address, age and occupation: a note should also be made of administrative details such as a treatment number.

Relevant medical history

There are a few items in a medical history of which one should be aware before prescribing a partial denture. Epilepsy may be cited as one example, as this condition might influence the design of a denture. However, a knowledge of the patient's medical history is particularly relevant to the preparation of a mouth in which periodontal therapy or any form of minor oral surgery is to play a part. The dentist needs to know of any heart or chest complaints or a history of rheumatic fever. The latter is of importance so that the patient may be protected against a bacteraemia which might lead to an endocarditis. Patients with an implanted hip prosthesis should also be protected from a bacteraemia which may result in an infection at the site of the implant. Precautions are also required for diabetic patients and those with a history of excessive bleeding on minor trauma. With the increasing use and complexity of drug therapy, the dentist must know of any medication the patient is already receiving so that he may avoid the use of a drug which reacts adversely to or potentiates the action of one already prescribed, or a drug to which the patient is known to be allergic.

Steroid drugs need to be boosted during the period covering an extraction, whilst anticoagulants must be reduced in a controlled manner. A knowledge of the drugs which a patient is taking may

Partial dentures

explain observations made during subsequent examination: a dry mouth may be associated with sedative or anticonvulsant drugs; the proliferation of yeast organisms in the mouth with the long-term use of antibiotics.

Special precautions must be taken in treating any patient who has suffered from a hepatitis of the Australian antigen B type.

Dental history

A broad outline of the patient's previous dental experience helps in assessing the patient's attitude towards treatment and indicates what the dentist may expect or particularly look for when examining the mouth. Enquiry should be made as to regular attendance for dental treatment, the reason for any extractions and a history of partial denture-wearing.

Examination

The examination is both extraoral and intraoral, visual and tactile. The findings of this examination may indicate further specific tests and the use of diagnostic aids.

Extraoral examination

The student will soon learn to observe and assimilate details of the patient's outward appearance without the necessity for a formal examination. Obvious gaps in the teeth are most easily noticed but other points to watch for relative to the provision of partial dentures are:
  Facial swellings.
  Facial asymmetry.
  The amount of tooth shown during speech.
  Disproportion between the jaws.
  Irregularity in tooth arrangement.
  A reduction in the vertical dimension of the lower third of the face.

Intraoral examination

Prior to carrying out the examination scaling of the teeth must be done, otherwise cervical carious lesions may be missed. There is much to be observed and hence much may be overlooked if an orderly sequence is not followed. The number and position of the

Clinical stage 1

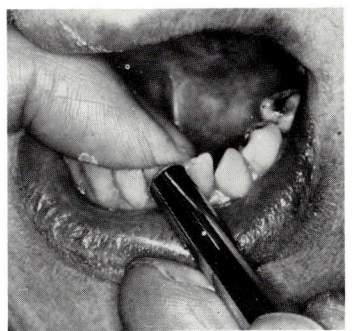

Fig. 1 Testing for fremitus.

teeth should be noted, together with the degree of drifting. In order to assess the relationships of the teeth one to another, it is necessary to view them in occlusion as well as in the customary open mouth position. The number and adequacy of existing restorations need to be assessed in addition to the detection of untreated carious lesions. Where the status of a tooth is uncertain, a vitality test is indicated.

The tissues supporting the teeth must be assessed clinically. Visual examination will reveal the adequacy of the patient's oral hygiene measures, the extent of any plaque and calculus deposits and the presence and degree of gingival inflammation. The use of a periodontal probe is necessary to assess pocketing around the teeth. Percussion of teeth aids in the diagnosis of a periapical lesion; the more gentle pressure of the mirror handle applied to the labiobuccal aspect of a tooth, with a finger placed on the lingual aspect, aids in the diagnosis of tooth mobility.

Fremitus, or the transmission of vibrations through the crown when tapped, is a normal finding with lower incisor teeth, where bony support for the roots is morphologically limited. In any other tooth, the phenomenon indicates the initial stages of weakening of the periodontal support (Fig. 1). Teeth exhibiting fremitus or the first signs of visible movement can usually be treated satisfactorily and subsequently play a full role in the retention and support of a partial denture. A tooth exhibiting rather more movement may be retained in the mouth (subject to treatment) if useful as a masticatory unit. However, it should be splinted by the partial denture and recognised as a tooth of poor prognosis and not employed to support or retain the denture. Teeth exhibiting 1 mm or more of movement should be extracted prior to the provision of the denture.

The mucosa of the tongue, palate and edentulous regions of the alveolar ridges may reveal signs of conditions requiring treatment. An inflamed or 'beefy' tongue can mirror an anaemia or vitamin deficiency rendering the mucosa of the patient insufficiently healthy to bear a partial denture. The palatal and alveolar mucosa may be inflamed with denture stomatitis; the condition must be resolved before accurate and reliable impressions can be obtained. The presence of a sinus in the mucosa might betoken a buried root; the mucosa of the sulci may bear a hyperplastic lesion caused by trauma from an overextended flange: these are examples of conditions which will require minor preprosthetic surgery.

The final element of the examination is represented by investigations designed to confirm provisional diagnoses formed during examination. A panelipse radiograph should be taken

Partial dentures

routinely of each patient and from this the need for more detailed radiographic examination can be decided (Fig. 2). Periapical and bite-wing radiographs of the mouth will show the degree of bone loss around the remaining teeth, periapical lesions on suspect teeth, buried roots, embedded teeth and interproximal caries.

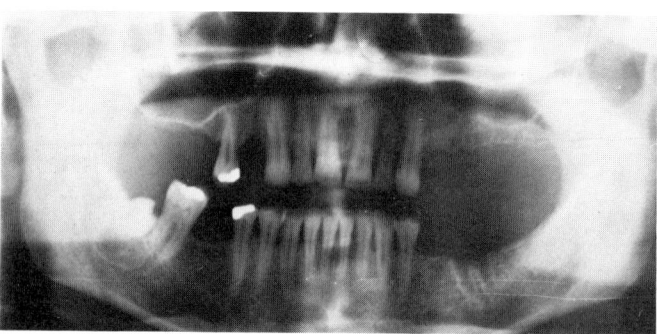

Fig. 2 An example of a panelipse radiograph used in the screening of a potentially dentate mouth.

A suspected anaemia and a candidal infection are two examples of conditions in which more specific tests may be required to confirm the diagnosis: a blood sample and a mucosal smear saliva culture being indicated in these two instances.

Provisional treatment plan

The examination will confirm whether or not the provision of partial dentures is the treatment of choice for the patient. If partial dentures are to be provided then a provisional treatment plan is made, designed to prepare the mouth for the new dentures. A typical provisional plan might include:

An extraction.
Periodontal therapy and oral hygiene instruction.
The restoration of individual teeth.

The term 'provisional' is used at this stage because the final design of the partial dentures can be decided upon only after the examination of study casts mounted on an articulator. Further mouth preparation is usually dictated by the design of the dentures (see pp. 53 *et seq*) and this is incorporated in the final treatment plan.

PRIMARY IMPRESSIONS

Objectives To obtain an impression of all the standing teeth and denture-supporting tissues of each jaw from which study casts may be prepared. The purposes of the study casts are:

Clinical stage 1

a To enable special trays and occlusion rims to be constructed if necessary.
b To examine the occlusion in detail on an articulator.
c By use of a surveyor, to plan the path of insertion of the proposed denture, arrive at a tentative design and plan any mouth preparation.

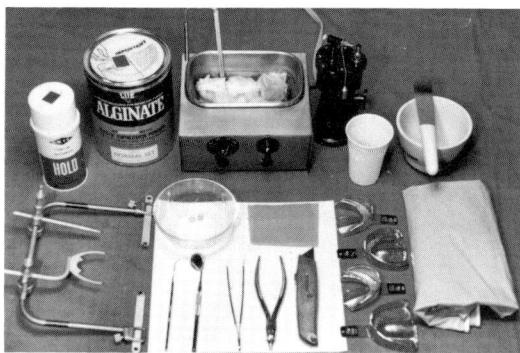

Fig. 3 Instruments and materials for registering primary impressions and jaw relationships.

Instruments and materials (Fig. 3)

1. Mirror, probe, tweezers.
2. Impression trays (Coe perforated Nos. 4, 7, 21 and 22).
3. Impression compound.
4. Water bath.
5. Adhesive solution.
6. Sharp knife (Stanley No. 199).
7. Hanau torch or pin-point flame.
8. Alginate impression material.
9. Mixing bowl and spatula.
10. Bowl for hot water.
11. Pliers.
12. Clean apron to protect patient's clothing.
13. Clean head rest cover and square for bracket table.
14. Mouthwash and denture bowl.

Procedure

Upper impression

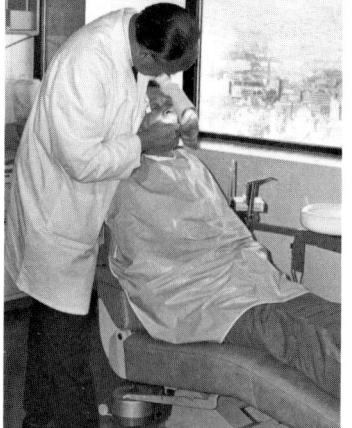

Fig. 4 The upper impression is taken standing behind and to the right of the patient. The patient's head is on a level with the operator's elbow.

On the patient's arrival:
1 Adjust the chair to a convenient working height (Fig. 4). Upper impressions are taken with the operator behind and to the right of

Partial dentures

the chair: the patient's head should be level with the operator's elbow.

2 Select the correct tray which will cover all the teeth in the arch (Fig. 5, A–C). The tray should leave a space of at least 3 mm between the flange and the buccal surfaces of the teeth. If the tray is of correct length but too narrow, use the pliers to bend the flange outwards. It will usually be too narrow in the posterior region.

3 A well designed stock tray may provide adequate support for the impression material in the sulcus and it should be tried in the mouth to check that no modification to the tray border is necessary. With many stock trays there may be a large gap between the border of the tray and the reflections of the mucosa in the labial and buccal sulci (Fig. 6, A). The flange of the tray should be extended into this gap (Fig. 6, B, C). This is best done with impression compound, which may be securely attached to the tray and when cold is strong and rigid. Wax is unsuitable to extend the tray because it will either come off the tray or bend and warp.

4 Use impression compound softened in the water bath and roll it out to the length and thickness of a pencil. Heat the edge of the tray flange and adapt the compound all around the edge. Make sure that it is securely attached to the outer aspect of the flange and is projecting beyond the edge. If the composition is too hard, flame it gently and dip it into the bowl of hot water. Do not put petroleum jelly on the composition.

5 Lift the patient's lip and hold out the cheek with your left hand, which is extended around from behind the patient. Rotate the tray into the mouth with the right hand. Seat the tray until all the teeth are resting on the base of its trough. The patient keeps the mouth open whilst the lips and cheeks are massaged to mould the composition into the sulcus.

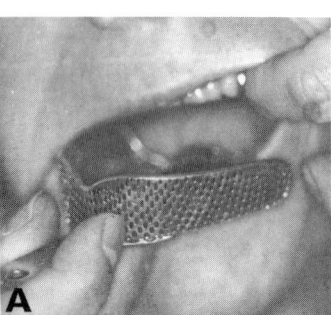 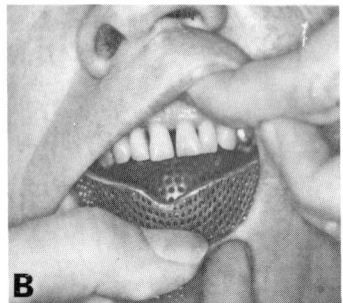 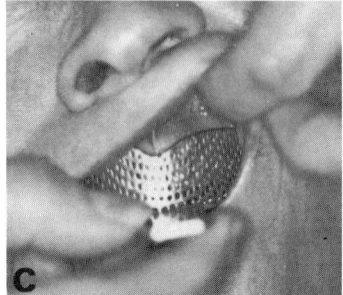

Fig. 5 (A) The left angle of the mouth is retracted as the tray is rotated into the mouth. (B) The upper lip is brought forwards to allow entry of the tray flange into the labial sulcus. (C) When the tray is in position, the border is checked to see that there is adequate extension into the sulcus.

Clinical stage 1

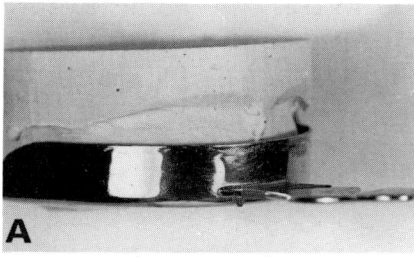
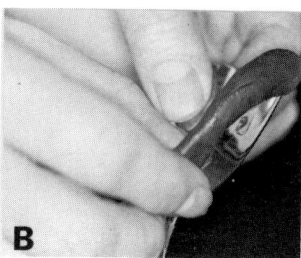
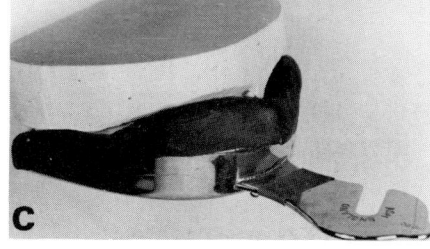

Fig. 6 (A) An underextended tray cannot support alginate impression material to register the sulcus correctly. (B) The underextended tray being modified by the addition of impression compound to the border. (C) The entire periphery of the tray has been modified to provide support for the impression material.

6 Lift the lip and check that the composition extends to the full depth of the sulcus. If it does not, note where it is deficient.

7 Remove the tray and add some more composition where indicated. This addition would be difficult if any petroleum jelly had been placed on the composition.

8 Now check the extension of the tray posteriorly. It must cover the last tooth and extend back to the hamular notch on each side. If it does not do so add composition to the posterior border in a similar manner.

9 Note if there is a large gap between the palatal section of the tray and the palate of the mouth. If there is it will be necessary to reduce this discrepancy, otherwise difficulty may be encountered introducing alginate impression material into the vault of the palate.

10 To add composition to the palate roll a small piece of composition into a ball about $1\frac{1}{2}$ cm in diameter (Fig. 7, A, B). Heat the palatal area of the tray and confine the addition of the composition to this zone. The material should not register an impression of the teeth when the tray is reinserted into the mouth.

11 Remove the tray. Chill the compound by immersing it in cold water. Check that the composition does not encroach on the teeth and trim the material away if necessary (Fig. 8, A, B).

12 It is essential that there be a sufficient space around the teeth for the inclusion of a good bulk of alginate material in order that there is no risk of distortion when the completed impression is

Partial dentures

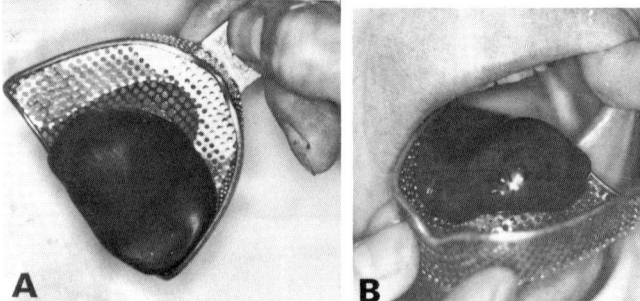

Fig. 7 (A) Impression composition is added to support alginate material in the palatal and edentulous ridge areas. (B) The tray with softened composition being seated in the mouth.

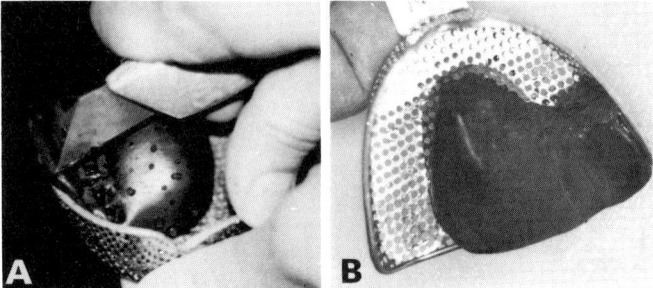

Fig. 8 (A) Any compound which has come into contact with standing teeth must be trimmed away. (B) The tray has been modified to give support in the palate and over a distal extension saddle and there is ample room around the standing teeth.

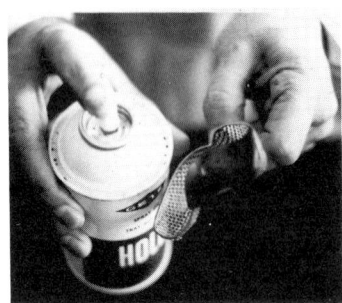

Fig. 9 An adhesive is applied to the impression composition and inner surfaces of the tray.

withdrawn. Use a sharp Stanley knife for trimming the composition. Blunt blades chip or distort the composition. A blade which is less substantial than that of a Stanley knife may break, causing damage to patient or operator.

13 It is now necessary to provide retention for the alginate material in the prepared tray. When using a perforated tray with impression composition, it is necessary to spray only the composition with a proprietary aerosol adhesive (Fig. 9). With trays which are not perforated the adhesive must be applied to the whole of the inner surface.

14 Many alginate powders are supplied in tins from which they are dispensed by means of a scoop. Where the specific gravity of the alginate powder is different from the filler, there tends to be a settling out of the heavier materials. It is for this reason that thorough shaking of the tin is recommended before the powder is measured. However, if the lid of the tin is removed after vigorous shaking, particles will be released into the atmosphere. An alginate whose

Clinical stage 1

particles are of nearly uniform specific gravity (Coe) or one in which the powder is dispensed in weighed sachets is to be recommended. A knowledge of the chemistry of the material will help prevent its abuse. Mix the alginate according to the manufacturer's instructions, taking care to use water at the recommended temperature. Spatulation should be vigorous, creaming the mix against the side of the bowl to eliminate unassimilated powder and produce an homogeneous material (Fig. 10).

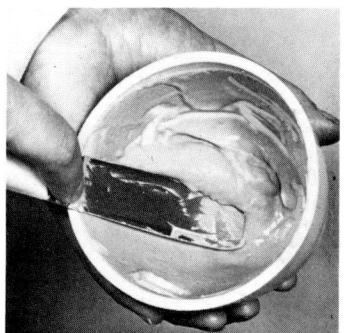

Fig. 10 Alginate is mixed by vigorous spatulation with the flat surface of the blade against the side of the bowl.

15 Load the alginate firmly into the tray so that no air locks exist beneath it (Fig. 11). It should not be necessary to fill the tray higher than the flange. With a napkin, remove any excessive saliva from around the patient's teeth. Place a small amount of alginate material from the bowl into the palate. This is best done with a spatula. Smear a little around the occlusal surfaces and into the embrasures. Hold up the lip and cheek with the left hand and seat the tray with the right. The anterior flange is raised into the labial sulcus and then the tray is raised posteriorly. In an attempt to assist the operator, the patient may open his mouth as wide as possible. This will result in the upper lip being so stretched that the tray cannot be placed in the labial sulcus. Once the loaded tray has entered the mouth the patient should be instructed to 'half close the mouth'. This will result in the lip becoming relaxed and it can easily be raised whilst the labial flange of the tray is positioned in the sulcus.

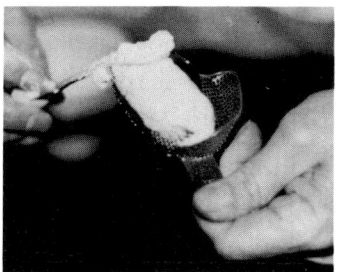

Fig. 11 The alginate material is loaded into the modified tray.

16 Once the tray is in place (Fig. 12) it must not be subject to pressure or any form of movement during setting of the material. Do not press on the tray and keep quite still. If the material is subject to loads as it sets it will be strained, and when removed from the mouth these strains will be released and distortion will result. Instruct the patient to tense the lip so as to bring the midline fraenum into relief and to move the cheek muscles to record the notches of the buccal fraenae. The tray must be left in place for $2\frac{1}{2}$ minutes. This will seem a very long time and therefore you must make sure that you use a watch or clock to check. The material will only then have achieved its full set and the strength and elasticity which will allow it to be removed from the undercuts around the teeth without any distortion. When you remove the tray do so with a rapid straight pull. Do not ease the tray out. The material is much more elastic under a sudden load.

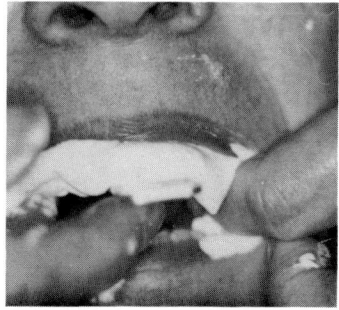

Fig. 12 The tray is seated in the mouth.

17 Check the impression (Fig. 13). Wash the impression under the cold tap to remove any mucus. Shake off excess water and examine the impression. A satisfactory impression:

14 *Partial dentures*

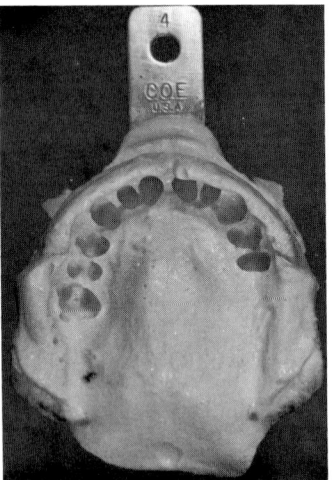

Fig. 13 The completed upper impression.

includes the whole of the sulcus and all of the teeth
has no bubbles or voids
exhibits no regions where the tray shows through.

Although alginate impression material is sufficiently elastic to be withdrawn from most tooth undercuts without distortion or tearing, the degree of undercut may sometimes be so deep that alginate will tear on removing the impression from the mouth. If this situation is encountered a stronger elastomeric material such as thiokol rubber or silicone may need to be used.

18 Cover the impression with a damp gauze whilst the lower impression is taken.

Lower impression

The height of the chair should be adjusted so that the patient's lower jaw is level with the operator's shoulder (Fig. 14) it is then possible to see easily into the mouth. After height adjustment, select a tray which will cover all the teeth and include the retromolar pad. Work from in front of the patient on his right side. The principles to be followed in the adaptation of the tray for taking the lower impression are the same as for the upper, the only difference occurring where there is a distal extension saddle. If this is the case, the procedure should be as follows:

1 Adapt the labial and buccal sulcus of the tray with composition as for the upper.

2 Adapt the lower anterolingual area to the functional form of the lingual sulcus.

3 Take a piece of softened composition $1\frac{1}{2}$ cm in diameter and adapt it to the posterior part of the lower tray and in that area which will cover the distal extension saddle. The tray will probably be

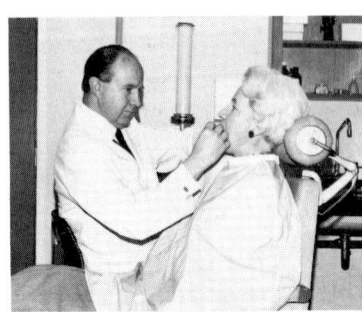

Fig. 14 The lower impression is recorded with the operator standing or sitting facing the patient, to the right. The patient's mouth is level with the operator's shoulder.

Clinical stage 1

short in this region and so the composition must be extended well beyond the limits of the lingual flange of the tray (Fig. 15, A).

The object is to obtain an impression of the saddle which is identical to the impression of this area in a complete denture. It should cover the external oblique ridge, the retromolar pad and the whole of the lingual sulcus, leaving room for the contraction of the mylohyoid muscle.

4 Adapt one side of the tray at a time. Seat the tray, requesting the patient to lift and protrude the tongue as the tray is seated. This will make sure that the tongue is not trapped beneath the lingual tray flanges and will allow the material to spread out underneath the tongue into the lingual sulcus. When the tray is seated, ask the patient to push the tongue hard up against the roof of the mouth. This will contract the mylohyoid muscle. Remove the impression and chill the composition addition on the one side and then complete the impression for the other side.

5 Remove any excess material from around the teeth and trim composition from undercut regions, such as the distolingual extension (Fig. 15, B, C).

6 Spray the composition with an adhesive material and prepare the alginate impression material.

7 Load the tray to the level of the flanges, with a coating of the alginate material covering the composition.

8 Rotate the tray into the mouth and position it above the tissues to be registered. With the left hand, draw the patient's lower lip forward and gently vibrate the tray into position. As the tray is seated, the patient's tongue should be raised and slightly protruded. When the tray has been seated into position, it should be held motionless whilst the patient is encouraged to make functional movements of the tongue, lips and cheeks.

9 When the alginate material has gelled, release the seal by retracting the cheeks and remove the impression with a snap action.

10 Rinse the impression and examine it critically (Fig. 16). All the teeth should be included, together with a complete registration of the buccolabial and lingual sulci. The impression should be free of air blows, particularly around the teeth and in the sulcus regions which might be required to carry the connectors of gingivally approaching clasps.

11 Cover the impression with a damp gauze. Do not rest the impression on a flat surface as this may distort the posterior part of the impression. Casts should be poured in the laboratory immediately after the patient's visit.

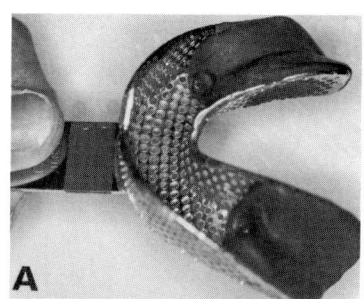
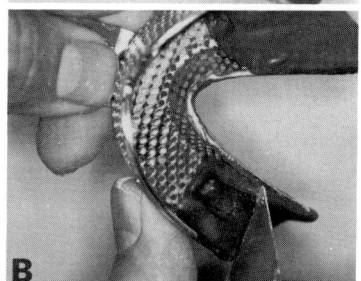
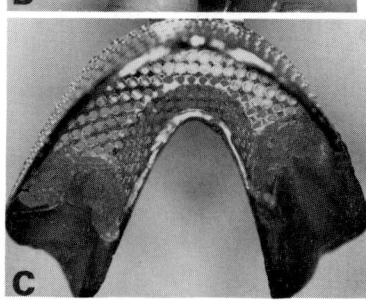

Fig. 15 (A) The edentulous regions of the jaw are recorded in impression composition. (B) Any impression compound which has engaged the abutment teeth must be trimmed away. (C) The modified lower tray ready for the application of an adhesive to the composition.

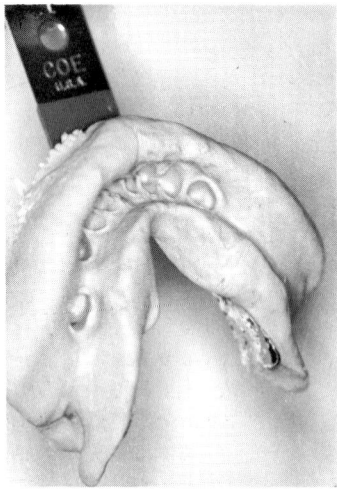

Fig. 16 The lower impression completed in an alginate material.

FACEBOW RECORD

A facebow record is necessary to relate the maxillary cast to the mandibular hinge axis on the articulator so that this position duplicates the relationship between the same structures in the patient.

1 The condylar hinge axis may be located with sufficient accuracy at a point 13 mm in front of the most posterior part of the tragus of the ear, on a line passing from the tragus to the outer canthus of the eye. These points should be marked on the patient's skin on each side of the patient's face.

2 The condylar slides are adjusted so that the readings on each side are equal, with the slides lightly touching the skin over the hinge axis points. The slide on the patient's left is then locked in position.

3 The fork is adjusted by bending to the approximate form of the upper arch. With the rod of the fork offset to the patient's right, a horseshoe of double thickness sheet wax is luted to the upper surface of the fork using sticky wax. The wax horseshoe should not be too bulky and not more than 2 mm wider than the buccopalatal width of the occlusal surfaces.

4 The wax is softened in a flame and the fork is pressed into position so that the occlusal surfaces of the upper teeth register in the wax rim.

5 The fork is held in position with the right hand whilst an assistant helps with the positioning of the facebow. It is more comfortable for the patient if the right-hand slide is fully withdrawn. As the facebow is positioned, the rod of the fork is passed through the clutch on the patient's right. When the bow is in position the right-hand slide is readjusted to the reading previously determined and locked in position.

6 The clutch holding the fork is tightened and the infraorbital marker passed through the clutch on the patient's left (Fig. 17). The infraorbital notch is located by palpation and the pointer directed towards the surface marking of the notch. The pointer clutch is tightened and the facebow removed.

JAW RELATIONSHIPS

Centric jaw relation may be defined as the most posterior relationship of the mandible to the maxilla at the established vertical dimension. It is therefore a relationship of bone to bone.

Centric occlusion is the maximum intercuspidation and/or planned contact of the teeth. In the subject with a complete natural

Clinical stage 1

dentition, the position of the mandible is usually slightly anterior to centric jaw relation when the teeth are in centric occlusion. When complete dentures are prepared it is usual to set the teeth in centric occlusion with the jaws in centric relation for reasons of denture stability. During the construction of partial dentures, it is necessary to decide whether to record centric jaw relation or that position slightly anterior which is dictated by the centric occlusion of the remaining natural teeth. The decision is frequently indicated by the circumstances. When there are insufficient posterior teeth to guide the mandible into a stable relationship with the maxilla, then the operator will endeavour to record centric jaw relationship and set the artificial teeth to centric occlusion on this basis. Where there are sufficient natural teeth to define centric occlusion then this position is used as the basis for the prosthetic reconstruction. The path of closure of the patient's mandible to the position where the natural teeth are in centric occlusion should be carefully observed. With the drifting of natural teeth into edentulous spaces even occlusal contact is frequently disrupted. As mandibular closure takes place in such a mouth the first occlusal contact may be an unstable one between two teeth only. A deflection of the mandibular path of closure takes place from this initial contact, and there may be other deflective or interceptive contacts before the teeth come to a position of centric occlusion. Such defects in occlusion, which may result in the patient experiencing pain from muscular spasm consequent to deflections in the path of mandibular closure, should be corrected by occlusal grinding before the provision of partial dentures. The modification of occlusal surfaces takes place as a planned procedure following the occlusal analysis of study casts mounted on an articulator. Fig. 18, A

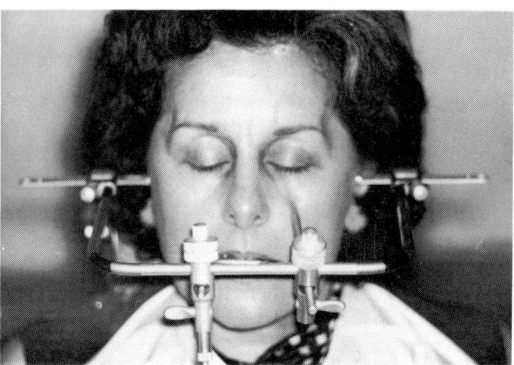

Fig. 17 The facebow assembly in position.

Partial dentures

shows the relationship of study casts at the first occlusal contact. Fig. 18, B demonstrates the centric occlusions achieved after deflective contact. Fig. 18, C demonstrates the occlusion planned and executed for the patient when the mandible closed in centric jaw relation.

Registering centric occlusion

When registering the position of jaw relationships there are three contingencies:

1 If there are sufficient natural teeth remaining it is unnecessary to make any record at all as the casts may be occluded using cuspal interdigitation as a guide.

2 If the centric occlusion is not quite positive but there are still several opposing teeth present, then it will be necessary to use a wax wafer record (Fig. 19). Form a horseshoe of two thicknesses of sheet wax from a prepared strip 8 mm wide and 80 mm long. Do not use an excessive thickness or an excessive width of wax. There should be no more than is necessary to cover the occlusal surfaces. An excess of wax predisposes to an inaccurate registration because the mandibular path of closure is readily influenced by a mass of soft wax and an eccentric position easily recorded. A useful alternative is provided by the so called 'bite wafer' manufactured for this purpose. One such material comprises a thin sheet of aluminium foil sandwiched between sheet wax. Another incorporates copper particles within the wafer itself. The inclusion of metal within the

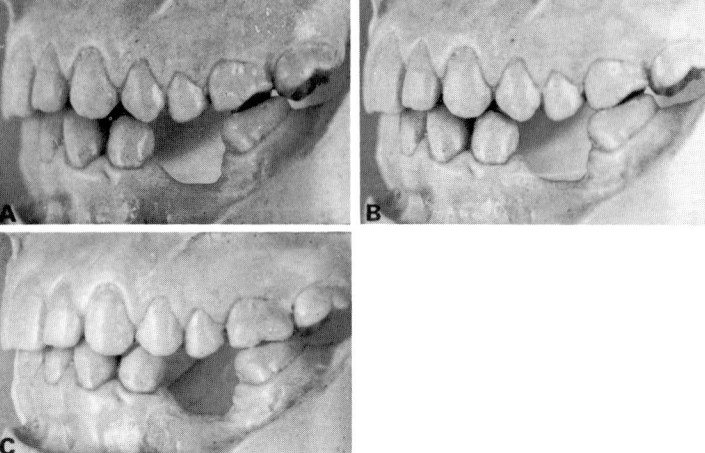

Fig. 18 (A) The first occlusal contact is between the disto-palatal cusp of the upper first molar and the occlusal fissure of the lower molar. (B) There followed a protrusive slide of the mandible to the position of centric occlusion. (C) After occlusal adjustment and the restoration of the upper first molar, this centric occlusion could be achieved without prior, deflective contact.

Clinical stage 1

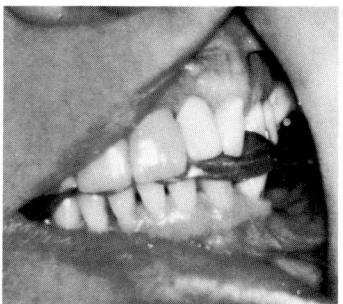

Fig. 19 A wax wafer being used to record centric occlusion.

wax ensures that the heat is adequately conducted throughout the mass. In order to ensure that the wax is evenly softened, it should be heated in a water bath.

The use of a quick setting zinc oxide/eugenol paste to record the occlusal relationship offers minimal resistance to jaw closure. The registration paste is spread on both sides of a thin gauze supported on the buccal and lingual sides by a framework which must be positioned free from interference with the occlusion (Fig. 20, A, B).

3 If there are insufficient opposing teeth, for example, where a bilateral distal extension denture is to be made, occlusion rims are necessary before the study casts can be accurately mounted on an articulator. If this is necessary then the patient will require to attend for an additional visit termed 1(a) in this schedule.

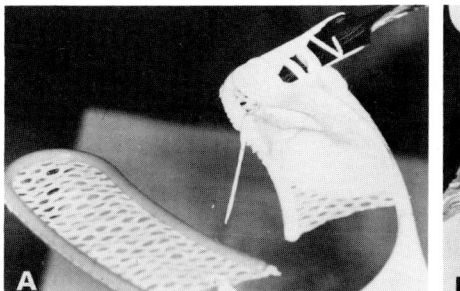 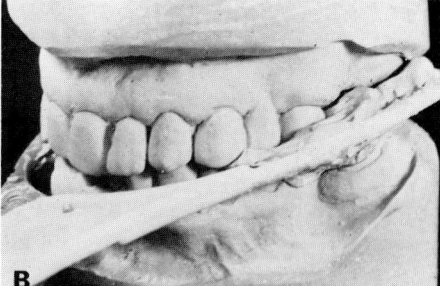

Fig. 20 (A) Applying registration paste to the framework. (B) Casts mounted in registration.

Clinical stage 1(a)

Registering centric jaw relationship

For this visit occlusion rims on self-cure acrylic bases are required. The construction of these is described in the first laboratory period. One of two situations may exist:
1 The patient's remaining teeth occlude at the correct vertical dimension.
2 Insufficient teeth are present for the patient to occlude at the correct vertical dimension.

A third possibility, that of a reduced vertical dimension due to occlusal attrition, may be present. In this instance, a form of prosthesis such as an overlay denture may be indicated to alter the occlusal vertical dimension. Such prostheses are not considered in this text.

Procedure

A *If the teeth occlude at the correct vertical dimension*

1 The patient is positioned comfortably in the chair sitting upright with the Frankfurt plane horizontal.
2 The upper rim is placed in the mouth and trimmed to the desired occlusal plane. Check that the rim does not interfere with the occlusal vertical dimension when the patient closes to centric occlusion.
3 Place the lower rim in the mouth and make the necessary adjustments, so that when the patient closes in centric occlusion there is an even contact of rims and natural teeth.
4 Trim $\frac{1}{2}$ mm from the height of the wax rims and cut 'V' shaped location notches into the wax. Prepare a single thickness wax wafer and, with the occlusal rims in the mouth, press the softened wafer on to the occlusal surfaces of the remaining lower teeth and the lower rim. Record the position of centric occlusion. Use the occlusal rims and wax wafer to check that the casts may accurately locate one to another before dismissing the patient. Alternatively the occlusal relationship may be registered using plaster of Paris (Fig. 21).

B *If insufficient teeth are present to indicate vertical dimension*

As the patient has no occlusal contacts to register the occlusal vertical dimension, then this must be determined by indirect means.

Clinical stage 1(a)

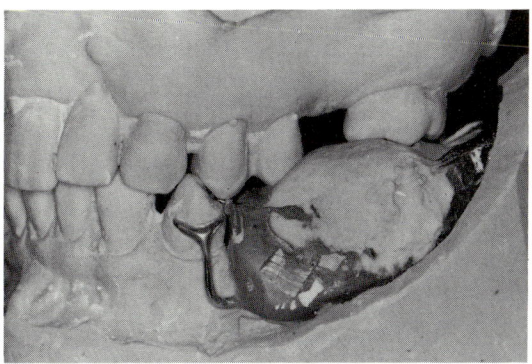

Fig. 21 The occlusal relationship being recorded using plaster of Paris on a wax occlusion rim.

1 Position the patient as recommended above in A.

2 Request the patient to lick the lips and then to sit with the lips resting gently together. The mandible should now be in the rest position.

3 Use a modified Willis gauge to record the distance from the columella of the nose to the menton (Fig. 22, A). (For placement beneath the chin, the sliding arm of the gauge should be shortened to half its original length.) This is the rest vertical dimension. Because the soft tissues are compressible and the angulation of the gauge to the face profile affects the reading on the scale, some operators prefer to make measurements with dividers between marks placed above and below the mouth on the mid line (Fig. 22, B).

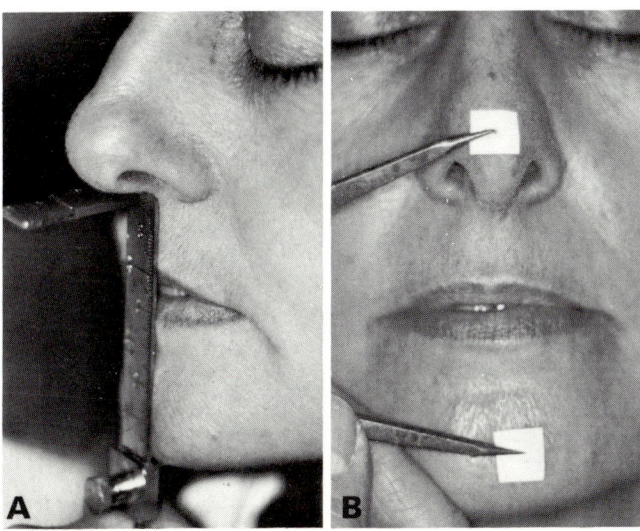

Fig. 22 (A) The use of a Willis gauge for the measurement of vertical dimension. (B) The use of dividers for the measurement of vertical dimension.

4 Subtract 2–4 mm from the rest vertical dimension. This represents an arbitrary interocclusal clearance (or freeway space) and the figure which remains represents the occlusal vertical dimension.

5 Proceed as in A above until the occlusion rims meet evenly at the predetermined occlusal vertical dimension. Record the jaw relation with a wax wafer.

Laboratory procedures 1

In this period casts are prepared from the first impressions and mounted on an articulator using the facebow record and the interocclusal record. The design and the material of denture construction is decided upon and any preparation of the teeth or the ridges which may be necessary. If difficulty was experienced in modifying the box sectional stock tray to obtain an adequate impression, then a special tray will be required.

Casting the impressions

These instructions apply to casting all alginate impressions. It is very important that the alginate impressions be cast as soon as possible after they have been taken, otherwise distortion may occur.

1 Rinse the alginate impression for 30 seconds under cold running water. This is to remove all traces of mucus. Shake the impression to remove excess water from the teeth. If necessary, blow this out with a gentle stream of compressed air.

2 Mix dental stone using 50 ml of water and 200 g of powder. (Powder/water ratio is 4:1.) Spatulate this thoroughly for 1 minute.

3 Vibrate the stone into the impression. Add the material in small quantities, vibrating it from one heel of the impression around to the other end. A mass of stone placed in the centre of the impression will not flow evenly and voids will be created in the cast. When the impression is just filling up with stone, put it aside and place the material remaining in the mixing bowl as a mound on a glass slab or tile and invert the filled impression onto it. Gently vibrate the impression down into the base. As it is very easy to distort unsupported sections of alginate, there are dangers in vibrating an impression down into a mass of mixed stone. An alternative method which may be recommended is to pour the anatomical section of the impression initially and to leave this to set. Then the impression may be inverted onto a base of new plaster without fear of distortion (Fig. 23). The most common fault with the lower cast is that insufficient material has been introduced around the heels of the impression.

4 Allow the stone to harden for 1 hour covered with a damp cloth. The napkin which covered the impression in the clinic will be quite

Partial dentures

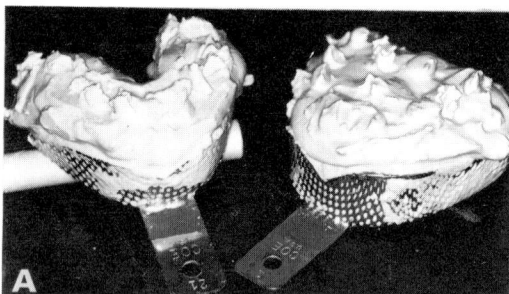

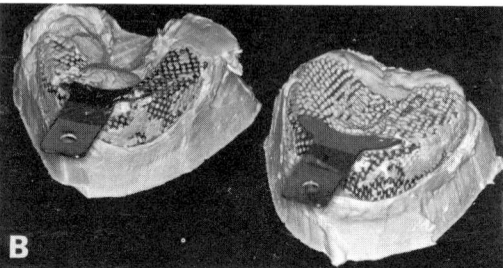

Fig. 23 An advised method of pouring a cast, without distorting the impression. The stone is initially introduced into the impression and left to harden (a). The tray may then be inverted and settled onto a stone base.

adequate. The impression should not be left on the cast for more than 1 hour.

5 If a perforated tray has been used, use a wax knife to cut off all the alginate which has extruded through the perforations. Immerse the cast and impression in hot water for 5 or 6 minutes to soften the composition. The impression tray should be removed from the cast without removing the impression material. The latter may be peeled from around the teeth. If the material comes off with the tray it is quite likely that teeth will break.

6 The cast is trimmed, care being taken not to remove the limits of the labiobuccal sulcus.

7 It is preferable not to handle the cast for another 24 hours, by which time the stone will be thoroughly hard.

PREPARATION OF OCCLUSION RIMS

Before a preliminary design can be arrived at it is necessary to survey the casts and mount them on an articulator. Wax rims on self-cure acrylic bases should be made on the study casts at this stage, if required (Fig. 24).

1 Block out tooth and soft tissue undercuts on the cast and coat the stone with a layer of alginate sealant.

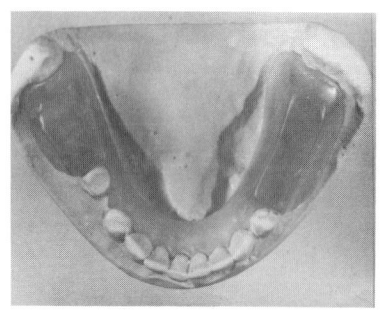

Fig. 24 A wax rim prepared on a self-cure acrylic base for the registration of jaw relationship.

Laboratory procedures 1

2   Prepare a semi-fluid mix of clear self-cure acrylic resin and pour this onto a glass slab which has been covered by a sheet of wet cellophane. Allow the surface of the acrylic to assume a matt appearance and cover with a further sheet of wet cellophane. Gently press a light glass slab onto the covering cellophane until the acrylic forms a sheet $1\frac{1}{2}$ mm thick.

3   Allow the acrylic to reach the dough stage of curing and remove the cellophane sheets. Press the acrylic sheet onto the baseplate area of the prepared cast and trim away excess material.

4   Place the cast and baseplate in an hydroflask for 10 minutes. When the acrylic resin is polymerised remove the base plate from the cast and trim the margins using a laboratory handpiece.

5   Apply sticky wax to the regions of the baseplate where occlusal rims are to be attached. Prepare the rims from hard modelling wax, warming the sticky wax before placing the rim in position. Trim the height of the wax rim to the occlusal level of the teeth on the cast.

6   Fluid wax is applied with a hot wax knife to fill the gaps between the occlusal rim and base on buccal and lingual aspects.

The clinical steps in recording the occlusal relationships have been described on pp. 20 et seq.

SURVEYING THE CAST

Objectives

1   To establish the path of insertion and guide planes for the denture.
2   To define those undercuts which may be used to retain the denture.

Procedure

As the term implies, the path of insertion is the direction in which the denture is introduced to its seating in the dental arch. Guide planes are provided by those faces of the natural teeth and alveolar ridge which lie parallel to the path of insertion; they may also be determined by the design of the denture framework which is constructed with parallel fitting surfaces forming a tangent to the maximum circumference of the teeth, and literally guide the denture along this path to its seating. Fig. 25 illustrates these features of insertion. The path of insertion is upwards and backwards, the mesial aspects of the distal abutment teeth and the alveolar ridge labially acting as guide planes. In multi-saddle dentures, the path of

Partial dentures

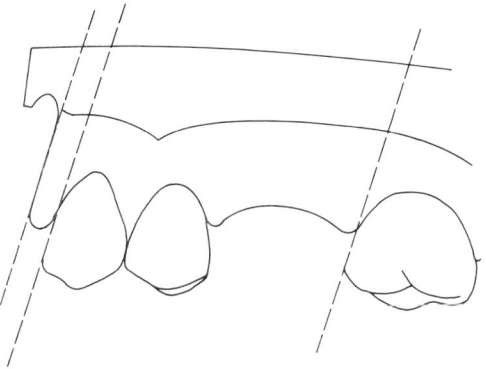

Fig. 25 Guide planes should be found parallel to the path of insertion. In this example, planes are formed by the mesial surfaces of the canine and molar teeth and the labial aspect of the alveolar ridge. It is unlikely that these three planes would exist in parallel without some preparation of the teeth.

insertion may be difficult to decide upon, but sufficient guide planes must be present or created to give the patient a well-defined line of insertion for the denture. In certain circumstances when selecting a path of insertion, it is advantageous to choose one which does not coincide with the potential vertical path of displacement of the denture during chewing. Fig. 26 illustrates how a denture saddle, introduced into a mesial undercut by an upwards and backwards path of insertion, resists vertical displacement.

The surveyor

In essence the surveyor consists of a vertically mounted chuck and a

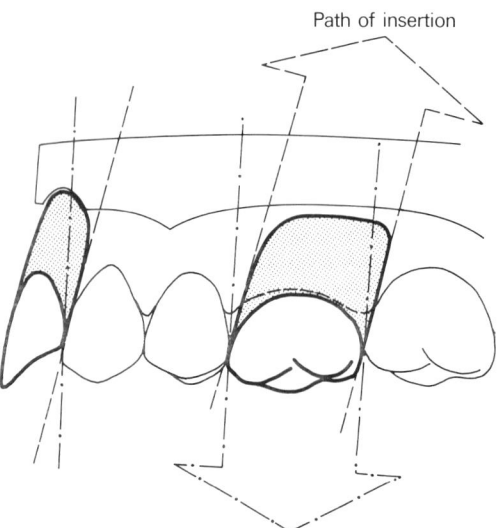

Fig. 26 By using an upwards and backwards path of insertion the denture can be made to engage undercuts, relative to the vertical path of displacement, on the mesial aspects of abutment teeth.

Laboratory procedures 1

table on which the study cast may be mounted (Fig. 27). The clutch is spring-loaded to move up and down in the vertical plane. The arm which carries it is designed to move to any position in the horizontal plane. The table is mounted on a universal joint, so that the orientation of the cast may be adjusted as required to the surveying instrument held in the chuck.

Surveying procedures

Mount the study cast on the table of the surveyor and the analysing rod in the chuck of the instrument. Start with the occlusal plane of the cast horizontal both anteroposteriorally and laterally. Place the analysing rod against the surfaces of the teeth and alveolar margins (Fig. 28). This procedure will give a preliminary indication of where the major undercut regions lie. The decision is then made as to which undercuts should be engaged by the denture base: as a corollary an initial path of insertion then suggests itself. Release the

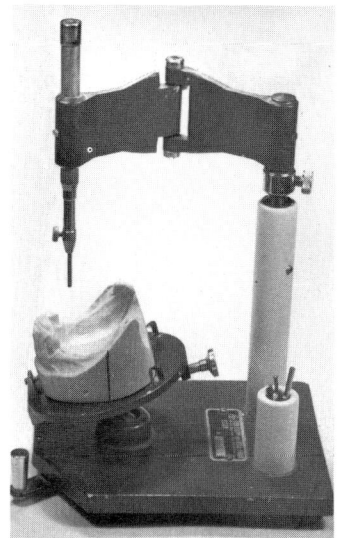

Fig. 27 Lower study cast mounted on the platform of the surveyor

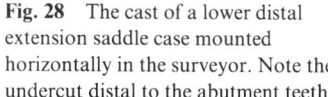

Fig. 28 The cast of a lower distal extension saddle case mounted horizontally in the surveyor. Note the undercut distal to the abutment teeth.

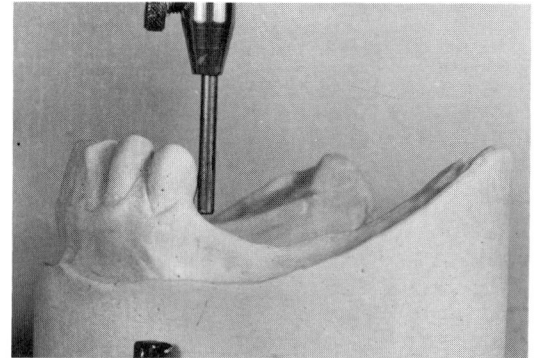

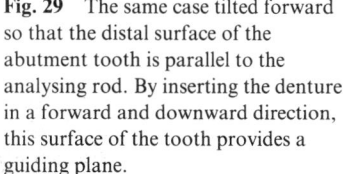

Fig. 29 The same case tilted forward so that the distal surface of the abutment tooth is parallel to the analysing rod. By inserting the denture in a forward and downward direction, this surface of the tooth provides a guiding plane.

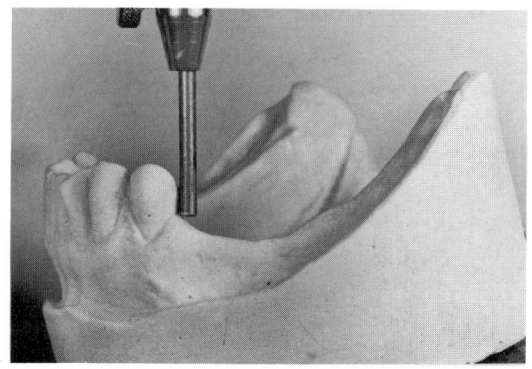

Partial dentures

universal joint on the surveyor table and adjust the orientation of the cast so that the analysing rod lies against possible guide planes. The position of the rod relative to the cast then indicates the tentative path of insertion. Lock the surveyor table and take the analysing rod around the cast again. Bearing in mind that, if necessary, minor alterations to tooth form may be undertaken with a sandpaper disc or diamond bur, make slight adjustments in the orientation of the surveyor table until the final path of insertion is decided upon. The student will soon learn to recognise standard paths of insertion for given situations:

Example 1   With the bilateral distal extension saddle in the lower jaw, distal surfaces of the abutment teeth form suitable guide planes, and the path of insertion is thus forward and downward (Fig. 29).

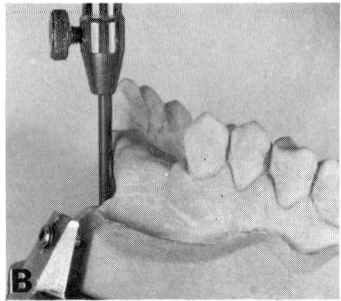

Fig. 30   (A) A maxillary cast of an anterior bounded saddle case mounted horizontally in the surveyor. Note the deep undercut beneath the labial alveolus. (B) By tilting the cast, all or most of the undercut can be eliminated. The denture will be inserted in an upward and backwards direction.

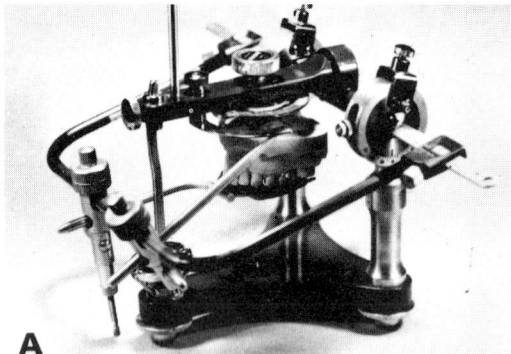

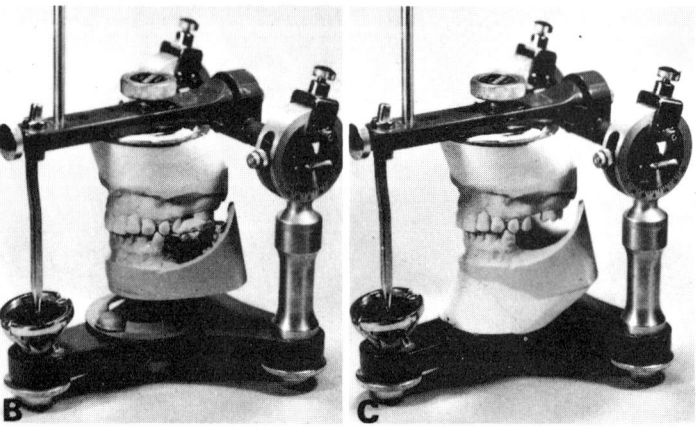

Fig. 31   Mounting the casts in the articulator. (A) By adjusting the extension screw in the universal joint holding the facebow fork, the infraorbital indicator is brought into contact with the infraorbital guide plane. (B) Having mounted the maxillary cast on the articulator, the mandibular cast is placed into position using the occlusal record. (C) The mounting of both casts is complete.

Example 2 Where there is an upper anterior saddle with four incisor teeth missing, the cast is orientated so that the analysing rod lies on the labial aspect of the alveolar ridge. The path of insertion is thus upward and backward with a flange engaging the undercut which exists relative to the vertical path of displacement. An additional advantage of this path of insertion is that the gap between the natural canine and the replacement lateral incisor teeth may be minimised (Fig. 30, A, B).

Replace the analysing rod with a graphite marker. Pass the marker around the teeth and alveolar ridges to produce a survey line. This line indicates the maximum bulbosity of these structures relative to the chosen path of insertion. Use the 0·25 mm and 0·50 mm undercut gauges to mark the depth of undercut on the buccal and lingual aspects of teeth which may be used for clasping.

MOUNTING STUDY CASTS

Procedure (Fig. 31).

1 The upper cast is mounted with the aid of the facebow record.
2 The lower cast is articulated with the upper in whichever way is suited to the situation; that is, either with or without a wax wafer or with record bases and rims. The casts should not be luted together with sticky wax on the teeth because it is not possible to remove the wax without damaging the cast. Instead, join the casts with old burs or stout wires luted to the bases.

Partial denture design

Before we discuss the stages necessary to design a partial denture, it is desirable to refer briefly to the subject of the classification of the partially edentulous mouth.

Classification of the partially edentulous mouth

Very many systems have been developed to classify the partially edentulous dental arches. Boucher observed 'apparently the systems were designed to simplify communications but variations between systems seem to defeat the purpose'. To be of use an acceptable system must immediately suggest the visual image of the partially edentulous arch and the simplest system which meets this criterion is that evolved by Kennedy, and this is the one which will be used in this text (Fig. 32, A–E). It relates the edentulous spaces to the abutment teeth.

There are four groups in this classification:

Class I   bilateral distal extension saddles.
Class II   unilateral distal extension saddle.
Class III   the unilateral bounded saddle.
Class IV   the anterior bounded saddle.

Classes I–III are modified by a number which indicates the number of additional edentulous saddle areas. Class IV has no modification.

In planning the design of any partial denture, a systematic approach is necessary. The four fundamental stages of partial denture design will now be discussed.

Outline saddle areas and plan support (Fig. 33).

The absence of a natural tooth is insufficient reason to replace it. Single tooth spaces tend to be reduced by the drifting of adjacent teeth which means that not only is the gap smaller, but that there are substantial proximal undercuts. These undercuts will require blocking out to allow insertion of the denture, leaving significant food stagnation areas. Thus, providing there is no tooth left occlusally unopposed, it may be wiser to leave the small space unrestored. Conversely, there is no point in restoring the small edentulous space when there is no opposing natural tooth or planned

Partial denture design 31

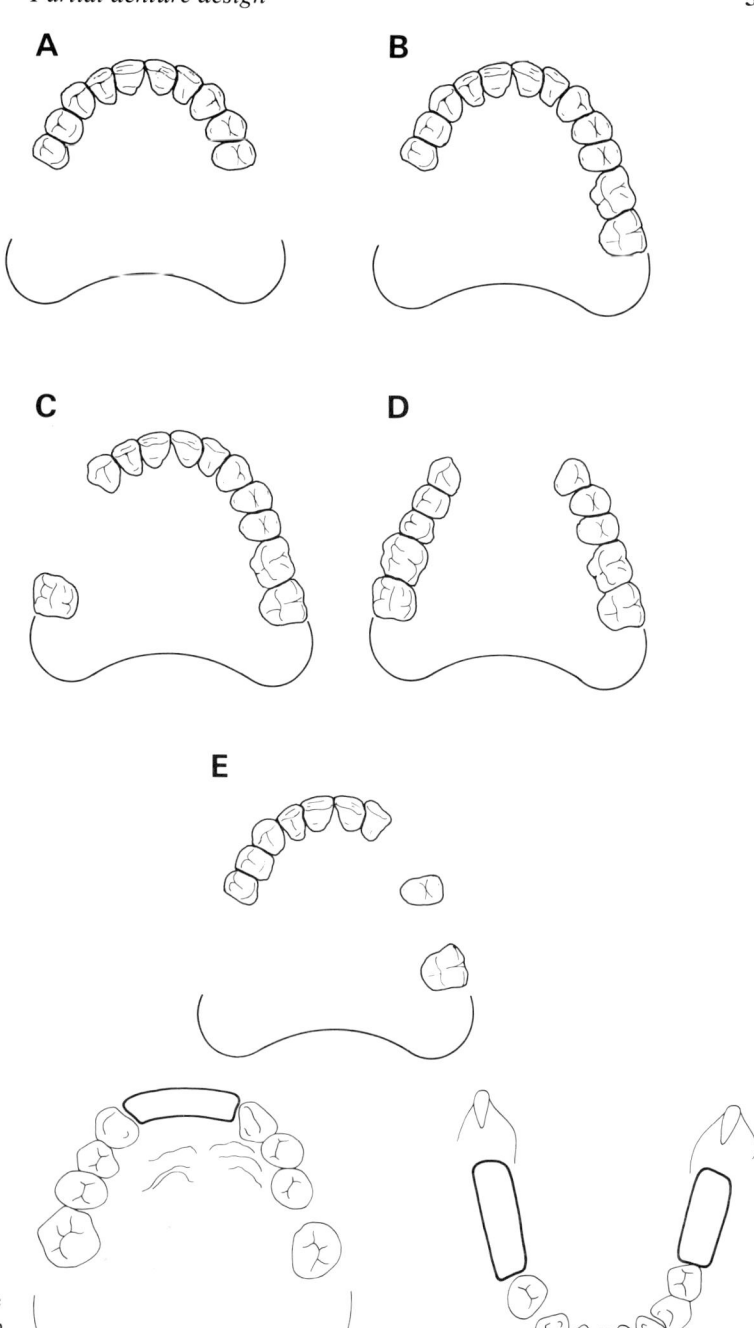

Fig. 32 The Kennedy Classification of Edentulous Spaces. (A) I Bilateral distal extension. (B) II Unilateral distal extension. (C) III Unilateral bounded. (D) IV Anterior, crossing the midline. (E) Additional spaces are indicated as modifications to the basic class—this example would be Class II, modification 2.

Fig. 33 The area of the occlusal table which is to be replaced is decided upon.

Partial dentures

replacement. Having decided which teeth require replacement, it is necessary to plan how forces generated by the musculature and transmitted through the denture are best opposed.

The masticatory load will be borne ultimately by the bone of the jaws. There are two ways in which the load may be transmitted from the denture to bone:

1 Through the natural teeth. The load passes to the alveolar bone as traction applied to the walls of the tooth socket by the periodontal fibres.

2 Where tooth support is not available, masticatory forces incident on the partial denture are transmitted to the bone as a compressive force by way of the mucoperiosteum.

When the mucoperiosteum must bear the masticatory load, the maximum area needs to be covered by the denture base in order to minimise the force per unit area. Where the saddle is bounded (i.e. with potential tooth support at each end), the masticatory load may be transmitted to these teeth by the agency of occlusal rests and overlays (Fig. 34). In such circumstances, the mucoperiosteum bears no load and the extension of the saddle is not so critical.

Tooth-borne dentures can sustain a greater clenching load than either mucosal-borne or tooth and mucosal-borne dentures. This is because the area of the periodontal ligament of a tooth is considerably greater than the area of mucosa which would cover the healed extraction site of that tooth, i.e. the support potential of the tooth-borne partial denture is greater than that of a mucosal-borne. Care must be taken not to overstress teeth selected to support a denture. As a generalisation, it may be stated that a tooth is capable of sustaining its own masticatory load and that of a further $1\frac{1}{2}$ replacement units. Factors which influence the support potential of a tooth include the number of roots, their size and form and the integrity of the periodontal tissue. First and second molar teeth and canine teeth have excellent support potential whereas the slender rooted lower incisors have a poor potential. A saddle carrying four

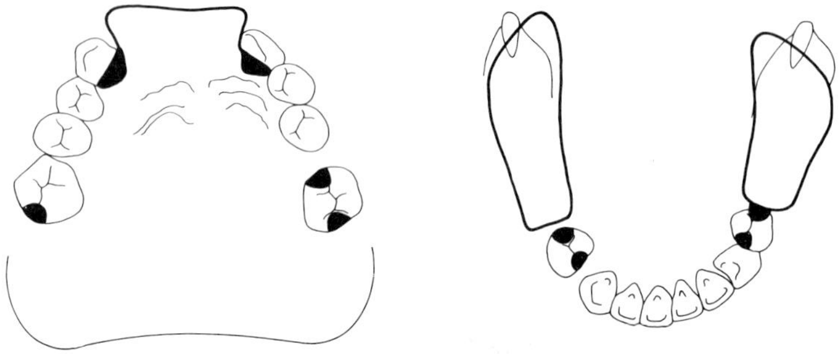

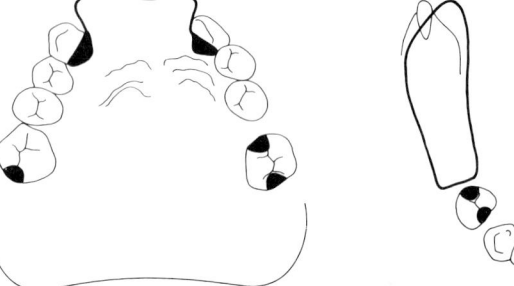

Fig. 34 The supporting elements of the dentures are designed. The upper denture will be principally tooth-borne, the lower, tooth and mucosal-borne.

Partial denture design

incisor teeth may be supported by two canine teeth (which are capable of bearing more than the 'average' additional $1\frac{1}{2}$ units of load). Conversely, a lower incisor abutment tooth should support less than $1\frac{1}{2}$ replacement units and if such a tooth is to be used in the support of a denture, it should be in conjunction with the use of other teeth in the intact part of the dental arch. These additional supporting teeth should not be too distant from the saddle and the connectors between their rests and the saddle must be completely rigid.

A tooth selected to support a denture needs to be periodontally sound with good supporting bone. Masticatory load transmitted from the denture should be directed down the long axis of the tooth. Occlusal rests should be positioned with this criterion in mind. The preparation of a rest seat is necessary where the rest might otherwise obstruct the occlusion or misdirect transmitted force. The positioning of rests need not be confined to the abutment teeth adjacent to the saddle. Additional rests placed on teeth in an intact part of the dental arch help to spread the load.

On occasion, teeth which have been treated periodontally but are below optimal condition are required for denture support. Such teeth should be splinted together wherever possible.

Tooth support is available only at one end of a distal extension saddle (Kennedy Classes I and II). Thus the maximum additional support must be obtained from the mucoperiosteum. The periodontal membrane of a supporting tooth yields far less to masticatory load than does the mucoperiosteum. The denture therefore needs to be designed to compensate for this difference in displacement of tooth and mucosa for any given masticatory load. There are two ways by which this may be achieved:

1 The saddle is made on a cast obtained from an impression which predisplaced the mucosal tissue, but not the teeth (e.g. the Applegate wax technique).
2 The tooth-borne and mucosal-borne components of the denture are flexibly connected to allow for independent movement of the mucosal-borne component (so called 'stress broken' designs). This is elaborated upon in Clinical Stage 3 (p. 75).

Select path of insertion and survey cast

The factors to be borne in mind when undertaking the procedure are:
1 The need to produce a definite path of insertion and withdrawal so that the denture may be placed and removed readily. This path

Partial dentures

should be at variance, wherever feasible, to the path of occlusal displacement of the denture in function, i.e. the path in which the denture might be drawn from the supporting tissue by sticky foods. The latter path is usually vertical.

2 The chosen path should allow for adequate retention, that is to say the survey of the cast must reveal adequate undercuts for clasps suitably positioned on the denture framework. Where no such undercuts exist some modification of crown form will be necessary.

3 The path of insertion should be chosen so that no unsightly gaps will be revealed in the mouth between replacement teeth and the anterior abutment teeth of saddles.

Guiding planes are derived from the path of insertion and are important in preventing the displacement of the denture along any other path. Contours of abutment teeth may have to be modified to achieve parallelism with these planes; alternatively, a plate design must be employed.

The path of insertion is selected using an analysing rod: when it has been decided upon, the path is marked on the side of the cast as a reference for any subsequent alignment (Fig. 35). The cast may then be surveyed.

Providing resistance to displacement away from supporting tissues

Retention is that quality of a denture which resists displacement away from the supporting tissues (Fig. 36).

Direct retainers

A direct retainer is a component of a partial denture which resists displacing forces acting along its path of insertion/withdrawal.

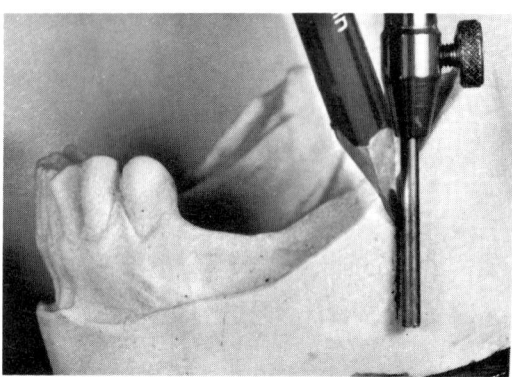

Fig. 35 The orientation of the cast on the surveyor table is marked with a pencil line drawn alongside the analysing rod.

Partial denture design

These may be extracoronal (clasps and precision attachments) or intracoronal (precision attachments only).

Wherever possible, clasps should be positioned in the denture design so that no axes of rotation exist. Where no suitable retentive undercuts exist on the crowns of abutment teeth, inlays may need to

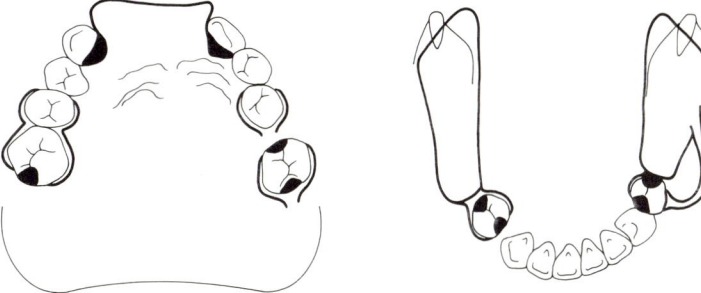

be prepared to receive ball-ended retainers. One of the purposes of surveying is to identify the areas of the teeth which are undercut relative to the axis of survey. Retention is provided by engaging an undercut surface with a flexible metal component. The extent to which the retentive element of a clasp will flex depends upon a number of factors:

1   The modulus of elasticity of the material of which it is made. Materials such as cobalt-chromium which have a high Young's modulus are stiff and therefore flex less than those such as wrought gold whose modulus is relatively low.

2   The further the terminal portion of the clasp is from its rigid attachment to the denture framework the more it will be flexed by a standard deflecting load.

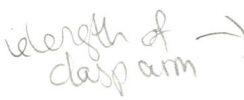

3   The shape and cross-sectional area of a clasp arm will influence the direction in which the metal can be most easily displaced and the extent to which such movement may occur.

From the foregoing, it may be deduced that when only a small undercut of 0·25 mm exists, a short clasp arm constructed in cobalt-chromium will be effective in resisting the displacement of the denture framework. With a large bulbous tooth such as an upper canine, if only a shallow undercut is engaged, the clasp will be visible; in this situation, therefore, it is necessary to engage a very deep undercut. A wrought gold clasp is usually used which approaches the undercut from the gingival margin and is thus much longer than a clasp which enters the undercut from the occlusal surface of the tooth.

It should be stressed that retention will only effectively resist the

Partial dentures

movement of the denture when it moves parallel to the direction of survey. In order to confine the denture to such a path of displacement, it is important that portions of the framework move along guide planes. Guide planes may be developed by careful discing of the tooth surface, by providing artificial crowns on abutment teeth which have been waxed up to parallel the desired path of insertion/withdrawal or by using a plate form of connector also constructed with its fitting surface parallel to the axis of survey.

A common fallacy which exists is to suppose that the bracing arm of a clasp (that on the opposite or reciprocal surface of a tooth) always serves to activate the retentive arm.

Reference to Fig. 37, A–E will help to explain why this is frequently not so.

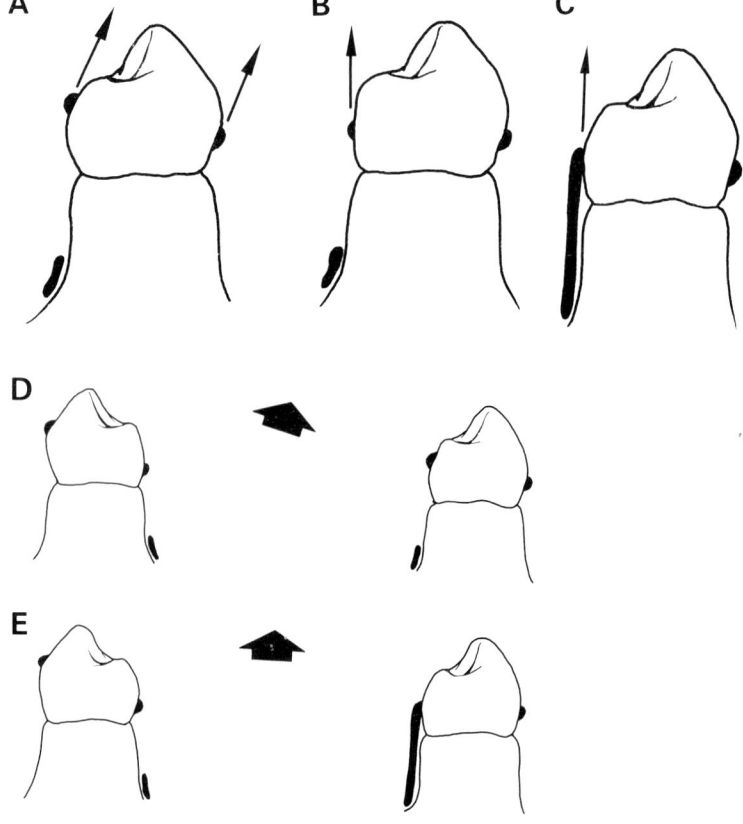

Fig. 37 (A) The tooth has been clasped after surveying about a vertical axis. Should the denture displace along the path indicated by the arrows, no resistance would be offered by the clasp. (B) The lingual surface of the tooth has been modified to provide a guide plane. This restricts the path along which the denture may be displaced and ensures that the functional arm of the clasp must be flexed over the bulbous crown before displacement of the denture may occur. (C) In this instance the guide plane is provided by means of a plate connector which restricts the path of displacement of the denture and so activates the clasp. (D) A cross-section of a skeleton framework in which a lingual undercut has been used on one side of the mouth and a buccal undercut on the other. Whilst the clasps will resist displacement in a vertical direction, movement may take place in the direction of the arrow without the clasps engaging any undercut. (E) By using a lingual plate connector on one side a guide plane is provided and the clasp arm is thus activated.

Partial denture design 37

Fig. 37, A represents a section through an abutment tooth on which has been placed a clasp which is part of a skeleton framework. The retentive arm of the clasp on the buccal surface of the premolar could move along a line which is a tangent to the tooth surface and, as parallel movement of the clasp arm on the lingual surface is not impeded, it does nothing to activate or reciprocate the retaining arm.

If the surface of the tooth were modified to provide a guiding plane on the lingual surface (Fig. 37, B) the path of displacement of the appliance would be controlled and the clasp would be rendered functional. The same effect is produced by a plate connector which is illustrated in Fig. 37, C.

What prevents displacement of the skeleton framework in many instances is the fact that the buccal surfaces of the teeth are engaged with the flexible retainer arms on opposite sides of the mouth. If it were necessary to use lingual undercuts on one side of the mouth and buccal undercuts on the other, as sometimes occurs, it is likely that the appliance would offer no resistance to displacement at all (Fig. 37, D). A plate connector which provides a guide plane resolves the difficulty (Fig. 37, E).

The design of clasp types is discussed in more detail at the end of this section.

At this stage the design consists of a number of individual components which must be joined together by connectors (Fig. 38). As the connectors may embrace a wide range of design, these are also considered at the end of this section.

Indirect retainers

It may prove impossible to avoid axes of rotation through clasp tips, particularly in Kennedy Class I and IV designs. In such circumstances, indirect retention becomes an important feature of design. An indirect retainer acts on the opposite side of an axis of rotation to the displacing force: its effect is to prevent movement of a saddle away from its supporting tissue. Indirect retainers usually have a further major function: examples include occlusal rests (support), baseplate extensions (support) and additional major connectors (the so-called 'continuous clasp' or Kennedy bar) or cingulum plate (Fig. 39, A–F).

Providing resistance to movement in the horizontal plane

A bounded saddle which is retained by clasps to both abutment teeth

Partial dentures

Fig. 38 The designs are completed by the positioning of major and minor connectors. The plate connector, or base, of the upper denture leaves gingival margins uncovered wherever possible. The lower study cast shows that there is insufficient depth of lingual alveolus to position a bar connector, thus a plate has been designed. The continuous minor connectors on the palatal aspect of the upper teeth not only integrate clasps and occlusal rests into the denture structure, but also brace the teeth against the retentive arms of the clasps. Similar functions are served by the lingual plate of the lower denture.

Fig. 39 The concept of indirect retention is explained in this figure. (A) Whenever a denture is retained by a two-clasp system, a potential axis of rotation exists through the clasp tips. (B) True vertical displacement is resisted by the clasp tip(a) and the denture base (b). (C) Displacement of the saddle is therefore rotational, around the clasp tips as they engage the bulbous part of the tooth. (D) Occlusal rests (c) or connectors (d), placed on the opposite side of the rotational axis to the displacing saddle, will help to retain the saddle in position by preventing the rotational movement. (E) The additional rests and connector have other primary functions, their positioning allows them to act as indirect retainers. (F) Where there is insufficient space for a lingual bar, a plate connector may be considered.

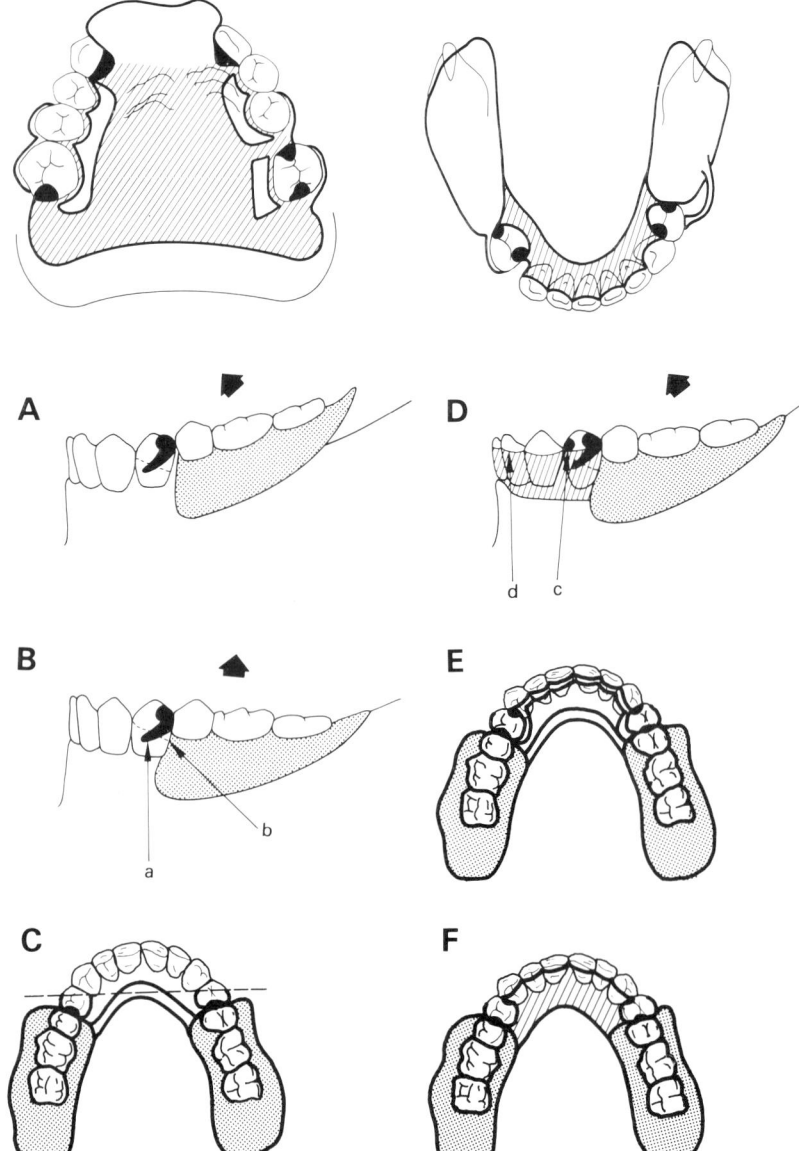

Partial denture design

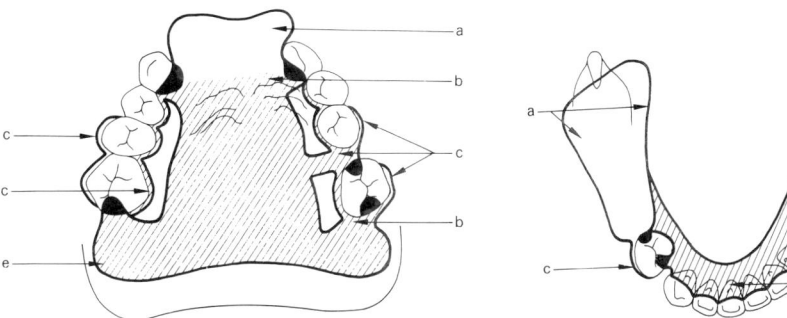

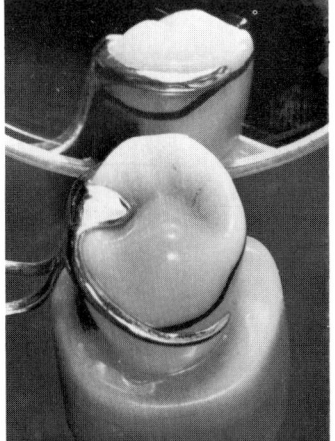

Fig. 40 Having assembled all the components of a partial denture to form a design, the resistance of this design to movement in the horizontal plane should be evaluated. There are several components which serve to brace the denture: (a) appropriate flange extension; (b) occlusal rest connectors; (c) clasp and connector elements; (d) lingual plate; (e) baseplate extension. Features bracing the denture laterally are on the left of each figure; and features bracing the denture anteroposteriorly are on the right.

Fig. 41 A C-form circumferential clasp with occlusal rest. The buccal arm engages an undercut whilst the lingual arm has a bracing function.

is braced anteroposteriorly by the presence of natural teeth and laterally by the retainers. Occlusally approaching clasp arms are more efficient in this respect than gingivally approaching ones. Distal extension saddles may be braced against posterior movement by engaging the mesial aspect of the mesial abutment with a rigid component (e.g. the minor connector of an occlusal rest) and by extending the saddle onto the retromolar pad. Cross-arch bracing should also be obtained from teeth on the contralateral side of the dental arch (Fig. 40).

By applying these principles to the case under consideration a design will have been arrived at and the modification of the natural dentition which will be necessary will have been decided upon. If it is necessary to modify the teeth, a new impression will be required. If stock trays cannot be readily modified to enable a good impression of the supporting tissues to be obtained, trays may need to be specially constructed.

Clasp design

So much has been written on clasp form and design that the student may readily become confused by minutiae; diverse terminology presents another hazard to clear understanding. The two major categories of direct retainers are clasps and precision attachments. It is convenient to consider clasps in four classes:

1. Circumferential (synonym: occlusally approaching).
2. Bar (synonyms: gingivally approaching; Roach).
3. Combination.
4. Embrasure.

Circumferential clasps

The arms of circumferential clasps embrace more than 180° of the circumference of the crown of the tooth, the retentive tips

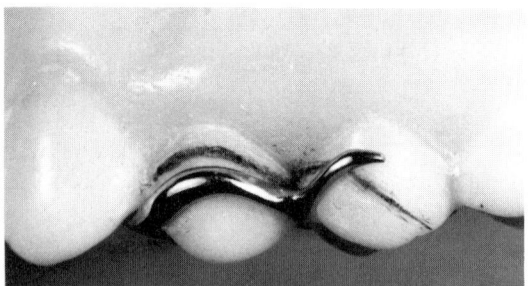

Fig. 42 An extended arm clasp. The arm extends across one tooth to a more favourable undercut on the adjacent tooth.

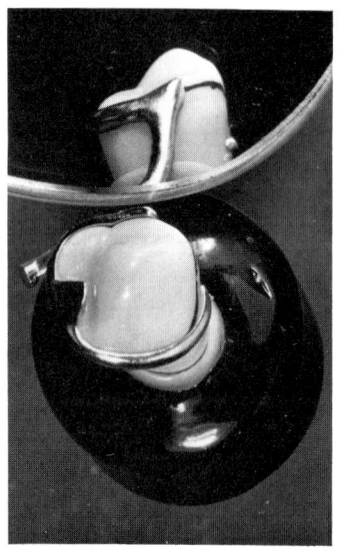

Fig. 43 A back action clasp. The connector is placed mesiolingually, whilst the undercut engaged is mesiobuccal.

approaching the undercut regions from the occlusal aspect of the survey line.

The simplest type of circumferential clasp is that having a *C-form* (Fig. 41). The minor connector for the clasp is positioned on the proximal aspect of the tooth, with the clasp arms extending into undercut regions distant from the connector. The clasp arm tapers from connector to tip so that the more rigid part of the arm, on the occlusal aspect of the survey line, may brace the denture against lateral movement.

Where there is no undercut on an abutment tooth and access to the undercut on the adjacent tooth is difficult from an occlusal approach, an *extended arm clasp* may be used. This clasp has the basic C-form, but the arms are extended across the buccal and lingual surfaces of the abutment tooth to the undercut of the adjacent tooth (Fig. 42).

Depending on the position of the connector relative to the clasp, the basic C-form shape appears in other guises. Fig. 43 illustrates a situation in which the minor connector is placed at the mesiolingual aspect of the tooth. The minor connector is usually joined to a major connector such as a lingual bar. The clasp arm curves around the tooth, supported distally by an occlusal rest, the retentive tip being positioned in a mesiobuccal undercut. A clasp which exhibits this feature of a retentive tip and connector positioned towards the same proximal aspect of the tooth is known as a *back action clasp*.

The *reverse back action clasp* is another variation on the C-form where a long connector is attached to the buccal arm of the clasp, the retentive tip of which is positioned lingually (Fig. 44). The connector is usually joined to an adjacent saddle of the denture. The problem in using back action and particularly reverse back action clasps is that it is difficult to make their connectors completely rigid. The *recurved clasp* (Fig. 45) has the retentive arm curved back upon itself to engage an undercut adjacent to the connector, which is

Partial denture design

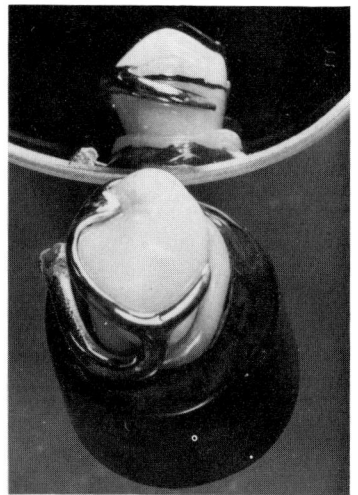

Fig. 44 A reverse back action clasp with a bucally placed connector. The undercut engaged by the clasp is lingually placed.

placed against the proximal aspect of the tooth. In theory, the increased length of the arm confers greater flexibility at the retentive tip, enabling a proportionately increased degree of undercut to be engaged. In practice, a good height of clinical crown is required to accommodate the recurve, which is particularly difficult to finish well in a cast clasp. Saliva tends to be held between the recurved arms by capillary action and this may lead to stagnation of food remnants predisposing to carious attack. The *encircling clasp* (synonym: ring clasp) is in the form of a single elongated arm which, as its name suggests, encircles the tooth to engage an undercut close to the position of the connector (Fig. 46). The connector is conventionally placed against the proximal aspect of the tooth. Because the bracing part of the arm (i.e. that part of the occlusal aspect of the survey line) is relatively long and is therefore difficult to make rigid, some writers suggest the positioning of additional connectors in the mid-buccal or mid-lingual aspect of the tooth.

These additional connectors give the clasp a superficial resemblance to a reverse back action clasp (cf.). They confer improved rigidity, but complicate the denture design and care must be taken to ensure that they do not encroach on the field of activity of the masseter or buccinator muscles.

Bar clasps

This form of clasp was popularised by Dr F. E. Roach in the 1930's. He himself used the term 'bar clasp', but the retainer became popularly known by his name. The synonym 'gingivally approaching clasp', arises from the position of the clasp connector, which is long and flexible, emerging from a saddle to cross the gingival margin of the abutment tooth and to end in a clasp head on the gingival aspect of the survey line. The length of the arm connecting the retentive terminal portion of the retainer to the denture framework may be varied, thus increasing or decreasing the flexibility of the retainer. Although the clasp rests passively against the tooth surface when the denture is seated, movement of the denture away from its support tissue causes the clasp to engage the tooth in the infrabulge position, conferring the required retention. This method of clasp function is sometimes known as 'trip action'.

The disadvantages of the bar clasp arise from the connector. Its flexibility may enable relatively large undercuts to be engaged, thus securing good retention, but the clasp has no rigid component to

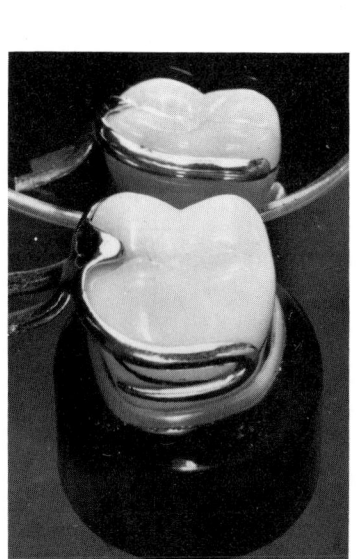

Fig. 45 A recurved arm clasp.

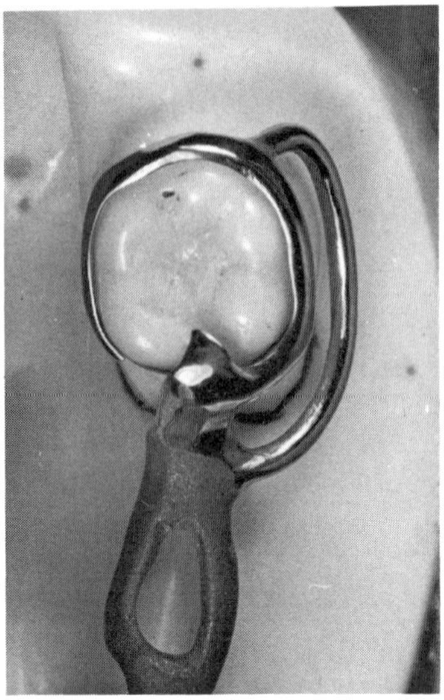

Partial dentures

brace the denture base against lateral displacement. The connector may also trap food. For both these reasons, it is unusual for a bar clasp to be used on posterior teeth. A group of bar clasps emerged, with various forms of clasp heads designed for the wide variety of survey line forms which could be encountered (Fig. 47, A–F). Recently there has been a tendency to simplify the clasp, reducing the amount of metal in contact with the tooth: this basic form is known as an 'I bar'. When a tooth exhibits no retentive undercut, as with a lower canine tooth, the terminal portion of this type of retainer may be made in the form of a ball and gains retention by fitting into a depression in a specially prepared cervical inlay.

Combination clasps

The combination clasp is one in which a bar arm forms the retaining element of the clasp, approaching the undercut across the gingival margin, whilst the tooth is braced on the opposing aspect by an occlusally approaching arm (Fig. 48).

Embrasure clasps

Fig. 46 An encircling or ring clasp with an additional connector to brace the structure.

It may occur that the crown of a tooth is of a less bulbous shape than is usually found or that it possesses a short clinical crown (as with children). In either case, there may be an absence of buccal and lingual undercuts on teeth which it is necessary to clasp. However, undercuts also exist interproximally, that is between adjacent teeth, cervically to the contact point. These undercuts may be exploited by the use of embrasure clasps, which may engage the undercut from the gingival or occlusal aspect.

The connector for the *occlusally approaching embrasure clasp* crosses the occlusal table in the interdental region and hooks into the infrabulge position from the buccal aspect. As these clasps are usually cast and have short connectors, they have little flexibility and therefore should not engage a great depth of undercut (Fig. 49). *Crib clasps*, such as the Adams (Fig. 50), are usually fashioned from 0·7 mm stainless steel wire and engage two interproximal undercuts. Their principal use is for orthodontic appliances, but they also find a use in retaining temporary dentures for children. These clasps should not be considered for permanent use on a partial denture.

The *gingivally approaching embrasure clasp* is a bar clasp with an 'arrowhead' ending. The point of the arrow is positioned to the gingival aspect of the contact point (Fig. 51); this type of clasp has the advantages and disadvantages inherent in bar clasp design.

Partial denture design

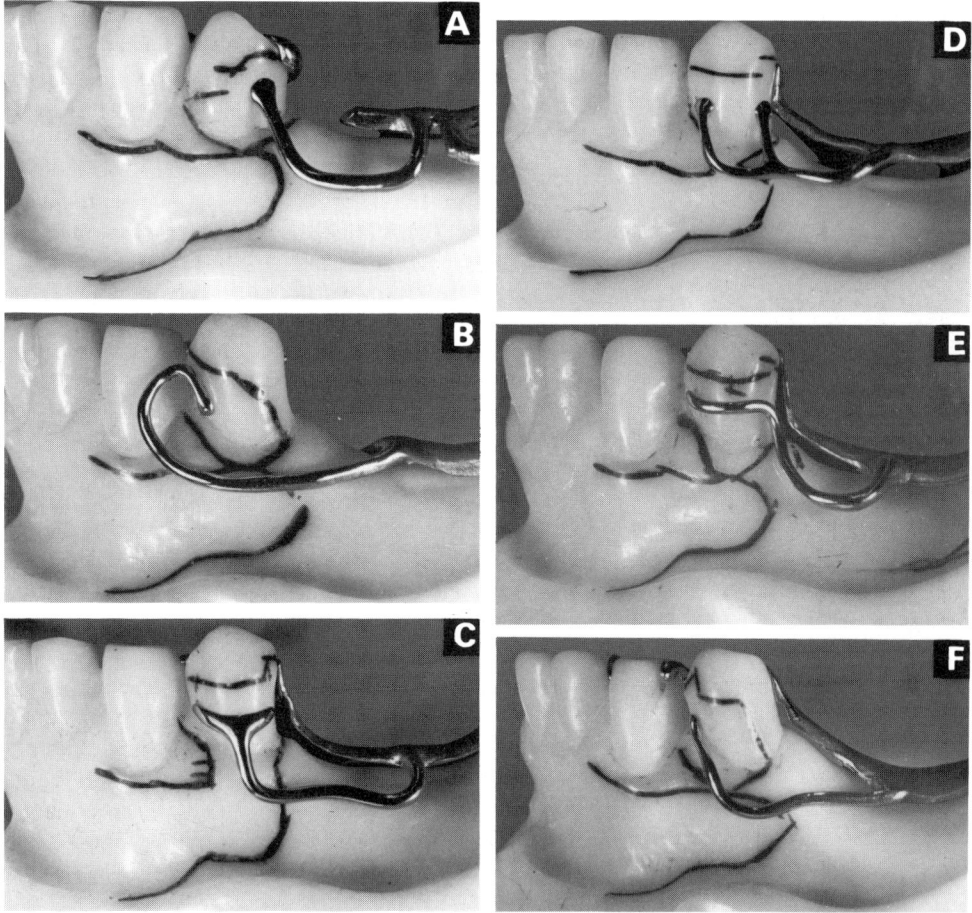

Fig. 47 A selection of bar clasps. The 'I' bar (A) is to be favoured for its simplicity and small area of tooth contact.

The foregoing is a brief description of the different choices of extracoronal retainers. There are, however, innumerable variations of clasp design, details of which will be found in prosthetic literature. In designing any retainer it is important that they satisfy the basic principles of design outlined below.

Principles of clasp design

1 More than 180° of the circumference of the tooth must be included. This may either be by the continuous contact of an

Partial dentures

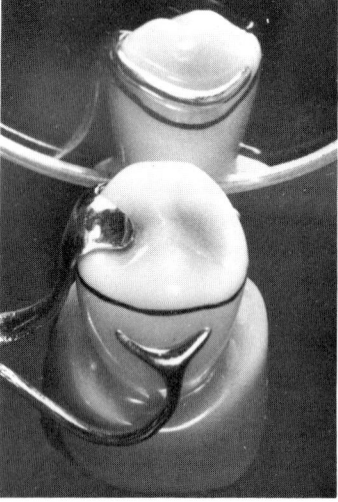

Fig. 48 A combination clasp. The retaining arm approaches the buccal undercut across the gingival margin whilst the bracing arm has an occlusal approach.

encircling clasp, or by the interrupted contact at two or more positions provided by the retentive terminal, occlusal rest and reciprocal in the case of a gingivally approaching clasp.

2   The denture should be designed to prevent movement of the clasp in a cervical direction.

3   The path of removal should be positively controlled by guide planes, if this is not achieved clasps should be bilaterally opposed.

4   In placing the denture the flexible terminal must not be displaced beyond its elastic limit and, when seated, it should not exert any pressure on the abutment tooth.

Design of connectors

A connector is a component of a partial denture which unites two or more other components. Those joining the saddle areas are usually referred to as major connectors and the others are known as minor connectors. Major connectors derive their strength in one of two ways:

1   From being made with a thick cross-section which imparts rigidity whilst, at the same time, minimising the area of tissue covered.

2   By covering a large area of tissue with a thin metal plate which derives its strength by being adapted to biplanar curves and by following the corrugations of the anatomy of the mouth. The former are referred to as bar connectors and the latter as plate connectors (Fig. 52, A, B).

The presence of a partial denture in the mouth interferes with the normal cleansing action of the tongue and leads to increased plaque deposition. If this is not removed by meticulous oral hygiene, inflammation of the gingivae and the formation of supra bony

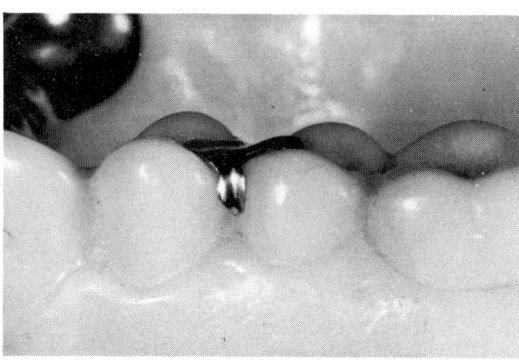

Fig. 49   Embrasure clasp approaching from the occlusal aspect.

Partial denture design

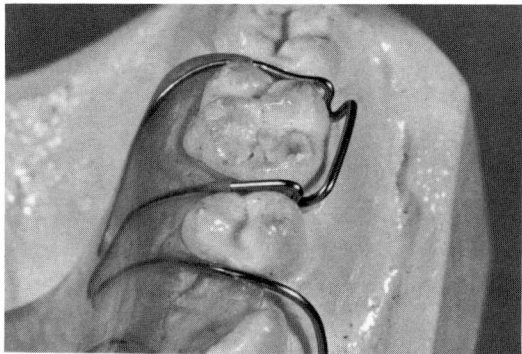

Fig. 50 An Adams crib clasp.

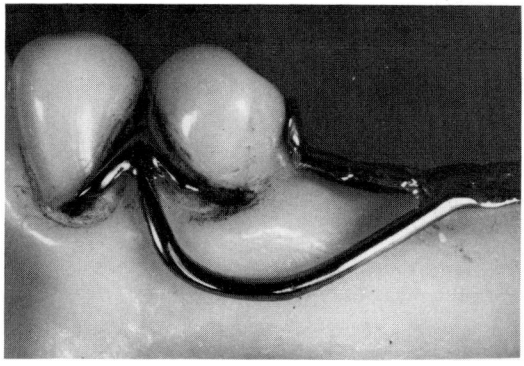

Fig. 51 A gingivally approaching embrasure clasp of the 'arrowhead' pattern.

pockets may result. As acrylic resin is porous and harbours plaque and bacteria, it is not an ideal material to place in contact with the teeth and its use as a base in partial denture construction is best confined to those situations dealt with in the Appendix. The desire to avoid the vulnerable gingival margin has led to the use of the so-called skeleton designs in which saddles and other components are united by bar connectors which avoid the gingival margins entirely. Unless the teeth have been prepared so that parallel tooth surfaces produce guide planes, dentures made to this design are likely to be unretentive as they may be displaced in a direction that differs from the axis of survey. Unless they have been adequately provided with support from the occlusal surfaces of the teeth, the bars themselves may transmit loads to the mucoperiosteum over a narrow area, thus causing tissue injury. A further difficulty may arise if the shape, thickness and position of the connector affects its tolerance by the patient.

Partial dentures

Indications for bar connectors

1 When adequate support can be derived from the teeth. Bar connectors should never be permitted to transmit masticatory loads to the supporting tissues. Therefore occlusal support is always necessary when bar connectors are being used (Fig. 53).

2 When it is desired to leave as large as possible an area of mucosa uncovered. Connectors must be designed and positioned to be unobtrusive: thus they should not be positioned across the middle of the palate and they should be designed in such a way that where the tongue is likely to pass over it the 'leading edge' of the connector is kept thin. Palatal bars which run parallel to the gingival margin should be positioned with a clearance of at least 0·5 cm from the gingival margin of the standing teeth. If a smaller space is allowed, the tissues tend to proliferate into it.

3 The labial bar is a form of connector to bear in mind where instanding lower teeth and the presence of distal abutments make it impossible to derive a path of insertion for a satisfactory lingual bar or plate. If adequate guide planes cannot be prepared lingually, the necessary blocking out of undercuts leads to food traps and a cramping of tongue space by the connector. A labially placed bar is free of such undercut areas (Fig. 54). However, it traverses a longer arc than its lingual counterpart and to retain rigidity is necessarily of thicker cross section.

Plate connectors can be made very thin and are less obtrusive. As they cover a wider area of the support tissues, they may transmit loads to the mucoperiosteum of the palate as well as to the natural teeth. By ensuring that the portion of the connector covering the lingual surfaces of the molar and premolar teeth are made parallel to the axis of survey, a precise series of guide planes is provided which enhance the activity of the retainers (Fig. 55, A, B).

As it is necessary to cover the lingual aspects of the standing teeth with the plate connector, there may be a danger that injury may be done to the gingival tissues. It has been shown that where space exists between the gingival tissues and the plate, there is a tendency for the tissues to proliferate, with the formation of supra bony pockets. This can be eliminated if it is possible to carry the metalwork to the gingival crevice, but this is only permissible when the denture is wholly supported by the natural teeth. If tooth support is not available, there is the possibility of the denture being displaced into the supporting tissues and thus stripping the gingival margin.

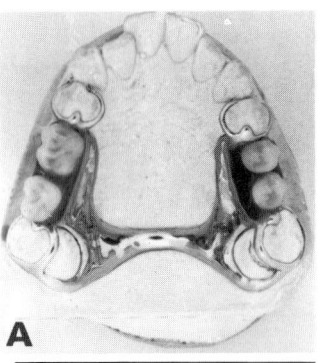

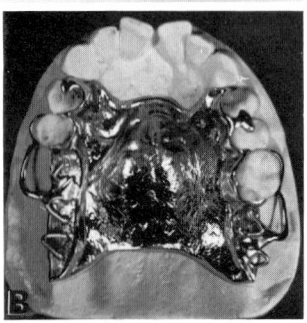

Fig. 52 (A) Two short tooth-supported saddles have been joined by means of a posterior palatal bar. (B) Although some tooth support has been used, the plate connectors provide additional support for the distal extension saddle on the unyielding mucoperiosteum of the palate. Guide planes also help to activate the retainers.

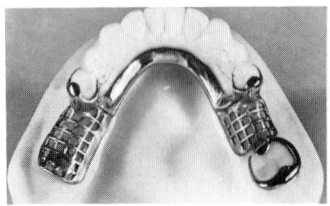

Fig. 53 The use of a lingual bar connector to join two saddles. Note the space required above and below the bar and the posterior clasping which prevents rotation.

Partial denture design

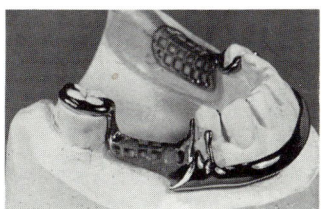

Fig. 54 A labial bar connector. Note the support provided by the teeth.

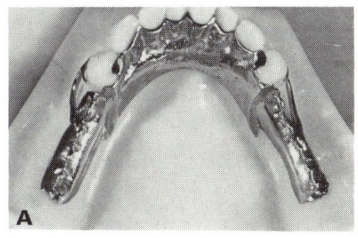

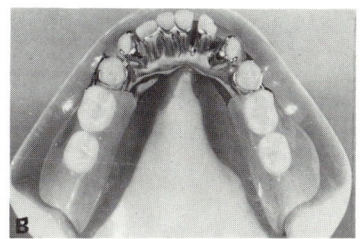

Fig. 55 (A) A lingual plate joining two extension saddles. (B) A split plate used in the presence of interdental space.

Fig. 56 A section through an upper tray made on a study cast to show the spacing required for an adequate thickness of alginate impression material.

Indications for plate connectors

1 When it is necessary to derive support from the palatal bone, the masticatory load can be spread over a wide area with this connector.
2 To achieve guide planes without modifying the crown form of the abutment teeth.
3 Where there is insufficient sulcus depth to recommend a bar connector.
4 When there is reason to suppose that bar connectors would be poorly tolerated because of their bulk.

Construction of special trays (Fig. 56)

Having considered the problems of denture design, it will probably be necessary to carry out some preparation of the standing teeth. This will either provide space for rests, provide guide planes or improve tooth form for retention. After this has been completed, new impressions will need to be taken. If perforated metal stock trays, modified as for the primary impression, conform fairly well to the arch form these will be used again. Where, however, the available trays cannot be modified satisfactorily special trays will be required.

1 The special tray for taking an alginate impression must be rigid, must cover all the teeth and denture-bearing area and extend into the labiobuccal sulcus and the lingual sulcus (for a lower tray).
2 The tray must be constructed so that there is sufficient clearance around the teeth. Undercut regions should be registered by a minimum thickness of 4 mm of alginate impression material if tearing or distortion is to be avoided on removing the impression from the mouth.
3 The flanges of the tray should be 1·5 mm short of the vault of the sulcus to enable a rolled border to be registered by the impression material.

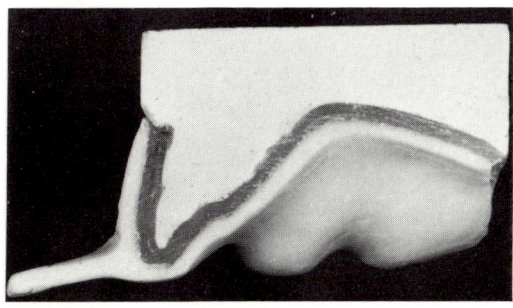

Partial dentures

4 The cast is prepared for tray manufacture by first waxing out all undercut areas. The area of the tray is then covered with two thicknesses of baseplate wax.

5 A sheet of self-cure resin is adapted to the wax spacer and allowed to harden.

6 A tray handle is attached in such a form and in such a position that it will not displace the lips, causing an inaccurate impression to be registered.

7 The tray should be perforated with a No. 10 round bur at 0·5 cm intervals.

Clinical stage 2

Objectives

1 To ensure that the mouth is in as healthy a state as possible before prosthetic treatment is begun.
2 To carry out any tooth preparation necessary to facilitate the design of a satisfactory denture.
3 To record impressions of the mouth as modified by **1** and **2**.

Instruments and materials (Fig. 57)

1   Mirror, probe and tweezers.
2   Special trays.
3   Handpieces, stones, diamond burs and sandpaper discs.
4   Occlusal indicator wax.
5   Articulating paper.
6   Alginate impression material.
7   Mixing bowl and spatula.
8   Clean apron.
9   Clean headrest cover and square for bracket table.
10 Mouthwash and denture bowl.

MOUTH PREPARATION FOR PARTIAL DENTURES

Provision of partial dentures represents the last phase of a treatment plan and the preparation of the mouth falls into two categories:
1 General care.
2 Specific preparation.

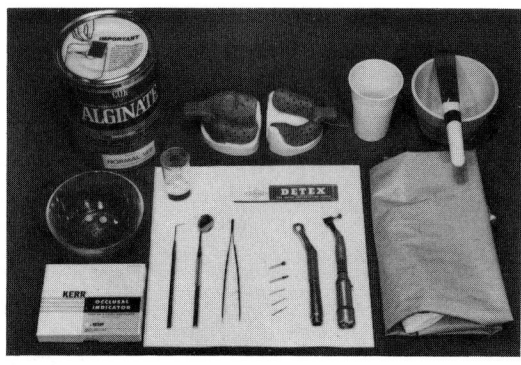

Fig. 57 Instruments and materials used in the preparation of the mouth and for the recording of secondary impressions.

Partial dentures

General care

1 Many generalised diseases have oral manifestations for which local treatment is ineffective. This is a wide topic outside the scope of the present discussion, but nevertheless one of which the operator should be aware.

2 Denture stomatitis may be present associated with an existing partial denture. The condition presents a livid inflammation of the mucosa under the denture base (Fig. 58). An accurate replacement

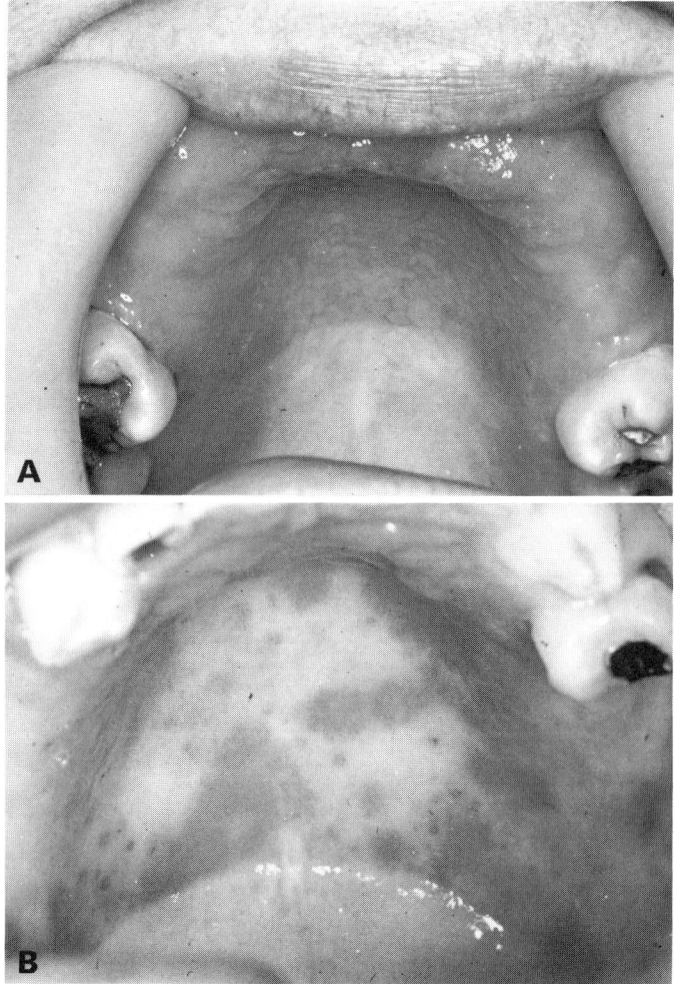

Fig. 58 Denture stomatitis presents as a livid inflammation of the supporting tissues with progressive fibrous change or hyperplasia. (A) Diffuse type, (B) discrete type.

Clinical stage 2

denture should not be made to an impression registering oedematous tissue, which must first be restored to a healthy condition by the following means:

a The patient should be encouraged to leave the denture out of the mouth. If this cooperation is not forthcoming, then the denture should be cleaned and lined with a tissue conditioning material (Fig. 59). The effect is to stabilise the denture and produce a resilient interface between denture base and mucosa. If the powder/liquid form of conditioner is used, then this should be replaced every 3 days, before resilience is lost as the plasticiser leaches out and the lining accumulates infected plaque.

b General oral hygiene measures and the use of hot hypertonic saline mouth baths should be instituted.

c Nystatin may be prescribed either in the form of 500 000 unit lozenges to be sucked twice each day (with the dentures out of the mouth) or as a cream applied to the denture base. Because nystatin has such an unpleasant taste amphotericin B (100 mg qds) is sometimes preferred although it may not be quite such an effective drug.

If the condition fails to respond to treatment with these fungicidal agents, it is advisable to check on the patient's serum iron level. If this is found to be below 14 μmol/l for a male, or 11 μmol/l for a female, a 6-week course of ferrous gluconate 300 mg tds should be prescribed. The patient should also be referred for a medical examination to elicit the cause of the iron deficiency.

3 The extraction of roots and teeth which are either decayed, of poor periodontal condition or malpositioned should be undertaken (see section on diagnosis).

4 The surgical preparation of hard and soft tissues to improve the

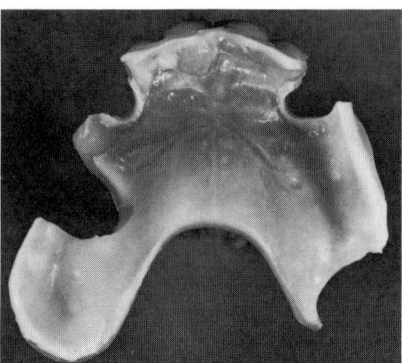

Fig. 59 The patient's ill-fitting old denture has been lined with tissue conditioner to promote healing of the damaged soft tissue.

Partial dentures

support area covered by the denture base. Two of the more common examples are the smoothing of a sharp mylohyoid ridge crest, which hazards the correct placement of the lingual flange of a distal extension saddle, and the excision of fibrous hyperplastic tissue associated with an existing ill-fitting denture. The reduction of a fibrous maxillary tuberosity may also be necessary to provide sufficient interalveolar space for the denture bases. Details of these and other procedures are considered by Howe (1971).

5   Any periodontal therapy which is necessary should be undertaken. Following oral hygiene instructions, the patient should demonstrate that he has mastered plaque control before the provision of partial dentures is contemplated.

6   Individual teeth should be in sound restorative condition and of good prognosis. In the latter respect, particular attention should be paid to root-filled teeth and those carrying post crowns. Where the restoration of a tooth is required, and it is known that this tooth is to be involved in the support or retention of a partial denture, then the operator should incorporate rest seats, undercut regions or guide planes as dictated by the provisional denture design (see below).

7   During the construction of the partial dentures, care must be taken not to introduce occlusal anomalies. It is therefore necessary for the patient to possess a path of mandibular closure unimpeded by deflective or interceptive occlusal contacts of the natural teeth. If, at the time of initial examination of the mouth, such contacts are suspected, then occlusal analysis should be undertaken (p. 17).

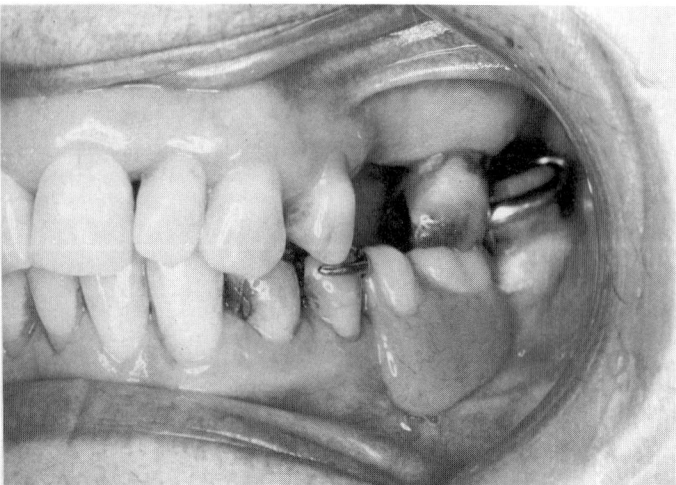

Fig. 60 A lower partial denture has been made without attention to the relationship of the natural molar teeth. The patient remains confined to 'hinge' movements of the jaw due to the obstructed occlusion.

Clinical stage 2 53

Specific preparation

All specific mouth preparations are planned on study casts mounted on an articulator when the denture is designed. Their site should be marked on the cast, so that the extent of the preparation is known when the patient returns for the ensuing stage of treatment.

Preparation of occlusal table

When examining the mounted study casts, the occlusal table should be visualised as it will be following reconstruction. If a natural tooth has been out of occlusal contact for a number of years then that tooth may well have overerupted. As a result, it will no longer conform to an acceptable occlusal table. Fig. 60 demonstrates the situation which develops if no thought is given to the occlusal table prior to providing a partial denture. The occlusion is completely locked in a 'centric' position as neither of the remaining natural molar teeth conforms to a satisfactory vertical position. The patient is unable to incise food with the anterior teeth because, when the mandible is protruded, the distobuccal cusp of the upper molar tooth occludes with the clasp connector on the lower denture giving rise to an anterior open bite.

Minor alterations in crown height may be affected by tooth preparation and subsequent full coverage crowns. Gross abnormalities (Fig. 61) may be corrected by extraction or by root canal

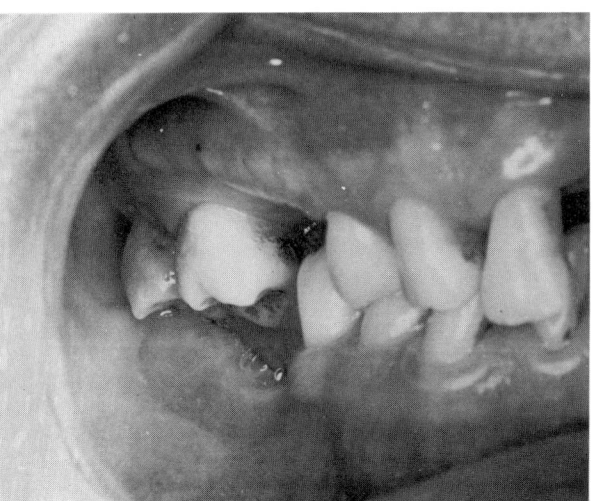

Fig. 61 Unopposed upper molar teeth have supra-erupted to disrupt the occlusal plane and obliterate the space required for the replacement lower teeth.

Partial dentures

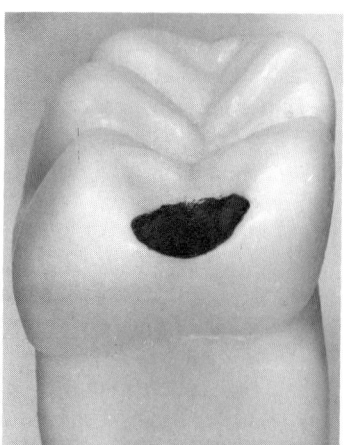

Fig. 62 A rest seat preparation on a molar tooth. The seat is within the thickness of the enamel; the dish-shaped profile is free of stagnation areas.

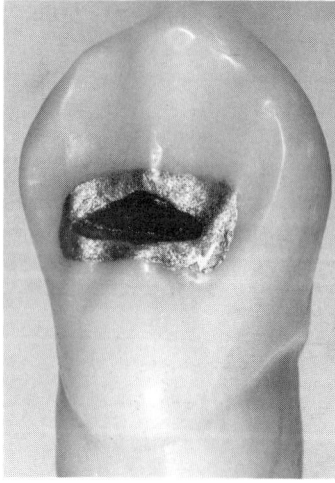

Fig. 63 A cingulum rest seat prepared in a canine tooth. Because an angular form is necessary to direct the load along the longitudinal axis of the tooth, it is desirable to cut the rest seat in a restoration positioned for this purpose.

treatment, following which the tooth may be de-coronated and the root face used as an overdenture abutment.

Modification of occlusal form

Seats are prepared for occlusal rests for one or more of the following reasons:
1 To smooth out enamel ridges and eliminate crevices beneath the rests.
2 To permit an adequate thickness of metal concomitant with the required strength of the rest, without creating occlusal interference.
3 To assist in directing the load applied to the tooth along its longitudinal axis. The form of the rest seat varies according to the material or tissue reduced in its preparation and the site.

In posterior teeth, the preparation of enamel should be undertaken with a round stone: the marginal ridge is first reduced and then the base of the cusps to widen the fissure or pit. The completed seat is dish-shaped and free of stagnation areas (Fig. 62). Preparation should be within the thickness of the enamel: if it appears that a greater depth would be required to eliminate occlusal interference, then the opposing cusp should be reduced. A rest seat prepared in an existing metal restoration should be confined to the restoration and be free of the margins. The preparation may be made with a tapered stone to produce a seat with a flat base and walls angled at 95°. The advantage of the wider, flatter base lies in the support offered by the rest seat, where potential stagnation areas are not a hazard. When anterior teeth are used for support, rest seats are positioned either on the cingulae (particularly with canines) or cut into incisal enamel. The necessity of preparing a rest seat which will direct incident forces along the axis of an anterior tooth makes the preparation of a cingulum rest without stagnation areas impossible (Fig. 63). Such rests should therefore be cut in restorations positioned for the purpose. Incisal rests are unsightly as the metal is difficult to mask, but they are used in some 'splinting' designs of lower denture. The incisal enamel should be prepared both mesially and distally to avoid stressing one aspect of the tooth's support structure. The axial walls of the preparations are made with a 5° taper and the lingual width of rest seats should be greater than the labial, to avoid placing preparations in an undercut relative to the path of insertion (Fig. 64).

Clinical stage 2

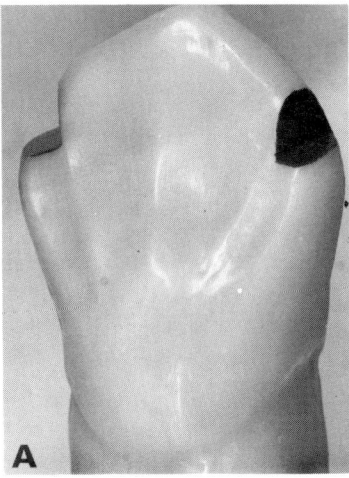
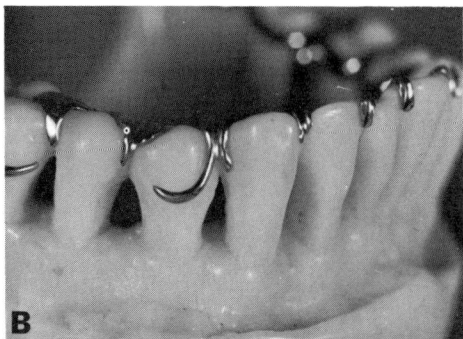

Fig. 64 (A) Incisal rest seats prepared on a canine tooth. These preparations are readily accessible for cleansing, but the rests are unsightly. (B) Multiple incisal rests on a denture designed to splint periodontally weakened teeth.

Modification of proximal and buccolabial form

The form of a tooth may require modifications of this nature for the following reasons:

1 Reduction of excess undercut at the proximal aspect of a denture saddle to reduce the food stagnation zones (Fig. 65).
2 To incorporate guide planes. This concept was discussed in the text dealing with design and selection of a path of insertion (p. 36). Reduction of the enamel thickness may be undertaken with a sandpaper disc. If more major modification of tooth form is required, then a full coverage metal crown is indicated.

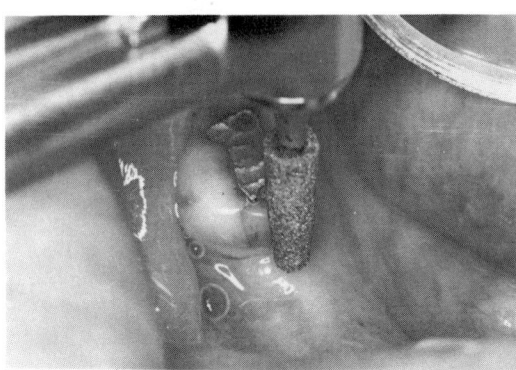

Fig. 65 The use of a tapered stone to reduce the mesial undercut on a molar tooth, thus eliminating a potential food stagnation area once the denture has been fitted.

Partial dentures

3 Where no undercut exists on a tooth from which direct retention is required, then this may be created in a specially positioned restoration. The most common example is the cervical inlay on a canine or first premolar tooth which carries a dimple, engaged by a ball-ended bar clasp (Fig. 66).

OBTAINING WORKING IMPRESSIONS

After the completion of any mouth preparation, it will clearly be necessary to take impressions of the mouth afresh. If perforated metal stock trays, modified with compound in the manner described on p. 10, conform fairly well to the arch form and will support the alginate impression material adequately, these will be used in preference to individually designed trays of acrylic resin. This is because the stock trays are rigid without being bulky; acrylic resin trays of the same stiffness tend to be bulky and more difficult to handle. The procedure for recording the impression is precisely the same as for the primary impression except that even stricter criteria must be applied before the resulting impression is accepted. If there is the slightest doubt about the acceptability of the working impression another should be taken. The consequences of a fault at this stage will involve the repetition of costly laboratory procedures as well as an additional clinical appointment.

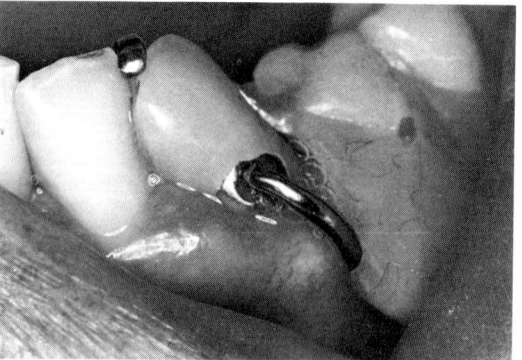

Fig. 66 A dimple has been placed in a cervical inlay and is engaged by a ball-ended bar clasp.

Laboratory procedures 2

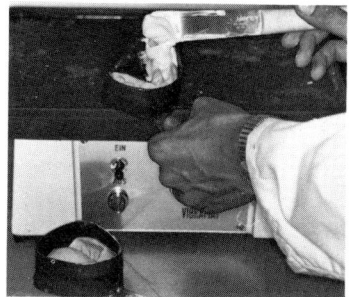

Fig. 67 The impressions are surrounded by boxing wax. The tray is held on the edge of a vibrator and stone introduced into one corner, so that the material flows onto the impression without voids forming in the cast.

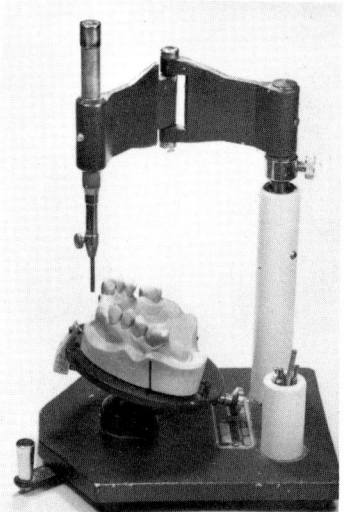

Fig. 68 The master cast mounted on a surveyor with the analysing rod paralleled to the angle of survey decided upon when the study cast was analysed.

PREPARATION OF THE MASTER CASTS

Both impressions should be boxed in to ensure that the form of the sulcus recorded in the impression is correctly reproduced (Fig. 67). A roll of beading wax is attached to the outer surface of each tray. With the upper impression, the beading is continued across the posterior border. With the lower, the beading continues around the lingual surface of the impression tray: the tongue space is filled in by a sheet of wax sealed to the beading wax. Boxing is completed by attaching sheets of boxing wax to the beading wax by means of a hot knife, to produce the mould into which the hydrocal slurry will be vibrated.

Surveying casts and outlining design

Designs have been decided upon after mounting and surveying the study casts and any mouth preparation to assist the construction of the dentures to these designs will have been carried out. The respective paths of insertion have been chosen and the master casts must be mounted in turn on the surveyor so that the analysing rod is parallel to the appropriate axis (Fig. 68). After checking for the presence of undercuts and guide planes, the analysing rod is replaced with a lead. The lead must have a straight edge and a bevel on one side of its tip (Fig. 69). The cast is surveyed with the bevel facing away from the point of contact of the lead with the cast. Both upper and lower limits of the undercut are marked. All those areas of the mouth adjacent to the final denture outline should be included. The leads used in the surveyor are very soft and the minimum contact pressure is required for the surface of the cast to be marked. The entire circumference of the abutment teeth should be included. There are occasions when surveying needs to be carried out about more than one axis: this is when the possibility exists for the denture to be displaced in more than one direction. The situation occurs with distal extension saddles, when rotation about a fulcrum provided by an indirect retainer gives a path of displacement which is not at right angles to the occlusal surface. Having obtained the survey line which shows the maximum circumference of each tooth relative to

Partial dentures

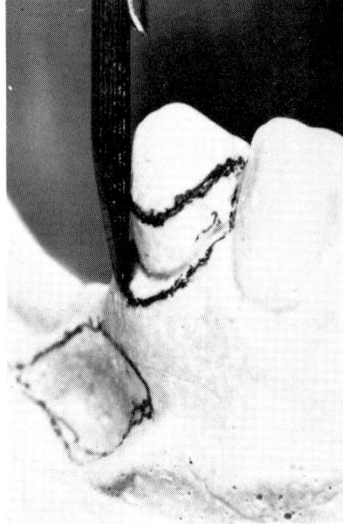

Fig. 69 The use of a graphite marker in the surveyor chuck to scribe the survey line. NOTE the bevel on the lead.

the chosen path of survey, it is now necessary to decide where the retainers are to be placed.

Use an undercut gauge to determine the position of the clasp tips in the undercuts, making reference to the detailed design plan (Fig. 70, A). The size of undercut gauge employed for each tooth to be clasped will depend on the material from which the clasp is to be made, the length of the connector and the design of the clasp (pp. 39 *et seq*). An alternative way of finding the undercut is to use the Scribt-o-meter which will measure the depth of any undercut portion of a tooth (Fig. 70, B).

Examples A short arm of a cast cobalt-chromium circumferential clasp (as on a premolar tooth) should engage a 0.25 mm undercut: the longer arm of a similar clasp on a molar tooth might engage a 0.37 mm undercut; whilst a wrought gold gingivally approaching clasp would engage a 0.5 mm undercut. A clasp which engages too deep an undercut will initially place an excessive pressure on the tooth. As the elastic properties of the metal are exceeded, the clasp will subsequently deform and may finally fracture. Mark the selected position for the clasp tip on the model with a sharp, soft coloured pencil (Fig. 71)

Modifying the master casts

1 Remove the model from the surveyor and block out gross

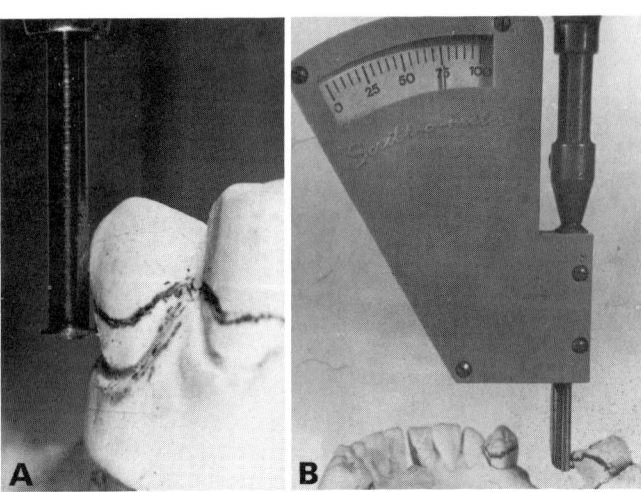

Fig. 70 (A) The use of a gauge to assess the depth of undercut. (B) The Scribt-o-meter for measuring the depth of undercut on a tooth.

Laboratory procedures 2

undercuts, in regions not involving the denture, with utility wax (Fig. 72). Such undercuts might be found in the labial aspect of the alveolar ridge where anterior teeth are standing. The blocking out of such undercuts minimises the possibility of splitting the duplicating gel on removal of the model.

2 Apply Wipla special carving wax to other tissue undercuts. The wax is applied with a small spatula (e.g. an Ash No. 5 instrument) which is warmed just sufficiently to cause the wax to flow into the required areas.

3 Replace the cast on the surveyor and place the trimming knife in the chuck. Trim the wax so that the undercuts are neatly blocked out cervical to the survey lines. All blocking out should conform to the chosen path of insertion. TAKE CARE NOT TO SCRAPE THE STONE CAST (Fig. 73).

4 Relieve the gingival margins to be crossed by bar clasps with Ash No. 4 soft metal foil (Fig. 74). The alveolar ridge area in the edentulous spaces should also be relieved with the same foil (Fig. 75): this ensures that when the metal framework has been cast there will be space beneath it for the acrylic base. Prepare locating shelves, in wax, for the arms of occlusally approaching clasps (Fig. 76).

5 Gently draw the base outline of the upper and lower dentures on the master cast with a soft graphite pencil (Fig. 77).

6 On the upper cast, lightly etch the outline of this base into the model (Fig. 78). The shallow dams thus formed slightly displace the underlying mucosa when the denture is placed in the mouth and help to prevent food debris from collecting beneath the denture base.

7 Where the pattern is to be sprued through the base of the refractory model, position a stud of the same size as the tip of the sprue former. This will make an impression in the duplicating gel into which the former may be fitted.

Preparing the investment cast

The modified master cast must now be duplicated in a refractory material and the denture framework is modelled in wax on this refractory cast. After spruing the pattern, it is completely invested in a casting ring and after the wax has been eliminated by heat, metal is cast to fill the void. Cobalt-chromium alloys are most commonly used for constructing partial denture bases as they provide great strength and resistance to corrosion in the mouth without resort to the expense of precious metals. As the metal contracts by 2% on cooling from its casting temperature, the mould into which it is cast

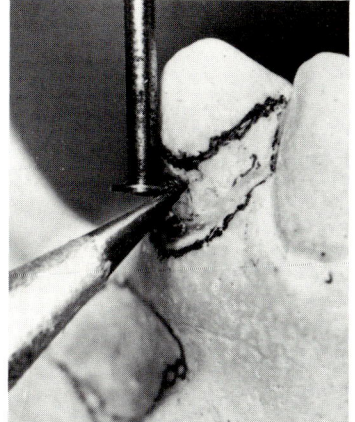

Fig. 71 Marking the required depth of undercut for a clasp. A soft, coloured pencil is used.

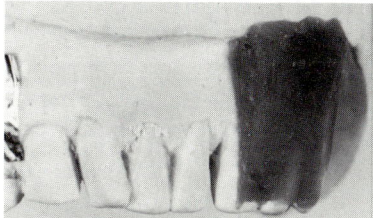

Fig. 72 Utility wax is used to block out major undercut areas, for example the labial sulcus, to minimise the risk of tearing the duplicating gel mould later in the procedures.

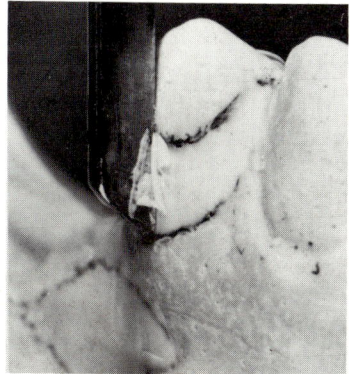

Fig. 73 The use of a trimming knife in the surveyor chuck to carve the blocking-out wax.

Partial dentures

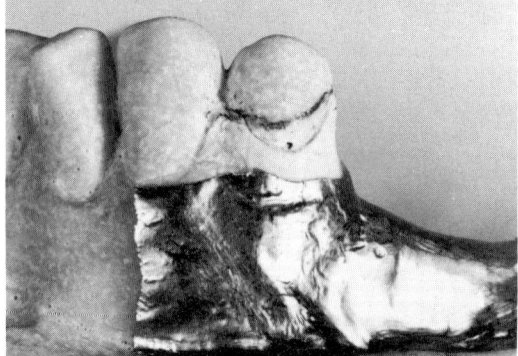

Fig. 74 The relief of the gingival margin to be crossed by a bar clasp connector.

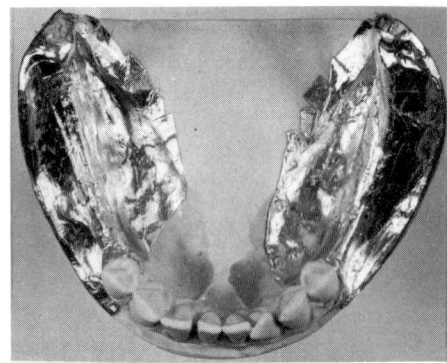

Fig. 75 The use of foil to relieve the saddle area of the cast.

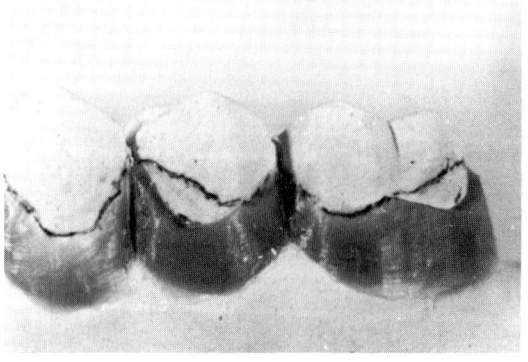

Fig. 76 Shelves prepared for the location of occlusally approaching clasp arms.

must be enlarged to compensate for this. This is achieved by the combination of the setting expansion of the refractory and the thermal expansion of the mould as the temperature is raised prior to casting. Thermal expansion is enhanced by the inversion of the silica allotrope of the refractory. Due to the high temperature to which the

Laboratory procedures 2

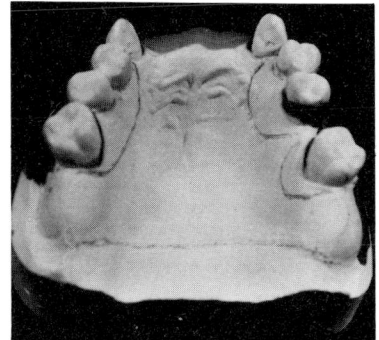

Fig. 77 The denture outline drawn lightly on the master cast.

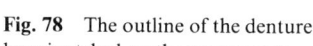

Fig. 78 The outline of the denture base is etched on the master cast.

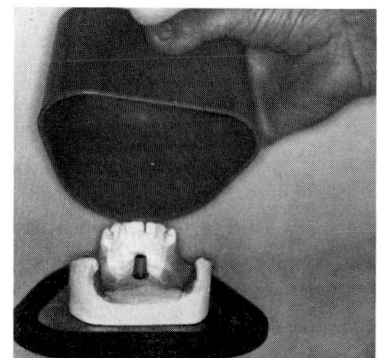

Fig. 79 Enclosing the prepared master cast in a duplicating flask. Note the stud positioned to aid location of the sprue former.

casting mould must be heated, the investment is made up of silica particles bound together by a silica gel (formed from ethyl silicate) or phosphate bond.

The latter preparation has largely superseded the silicate-bonded material due to the greater simplicity of this technique.

1 Soak the stone cast in warm water (40°C) for 20 minutes before duplicating to eliminate trapped air from the pores of the cast.

2 Stand the prepared cast on the base of a plastic duplicating flask and cover with the flask (Fig. 79). Pour duplicating agar at 52°C from the thermostatically controlled vat through one hole of the flask until it is full (Fig. 80). Bench cool the flask for 40 minutes transferring it to a water-cooled tray for a further 20 minutes.

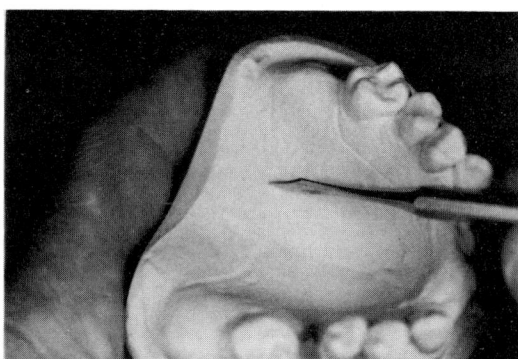

3 When the duplicating medium has gelled, trim away excess gel from the pouring holes and invert the flask. Remove the base of the flask and trim away sufficient gel from the base of the model to permit the cast to be levered gently from the gel (Fig. 81). Blow away moisture from the mould with a gentle stream of compressed air and examine.

4 If the mould is satisfactory, position the sprue former in the location prepared by the acrylic stud (Fig. 82).

5 Place 150 g of phosphate-bonded refractory material in a mixing bowl with 13 ml of water and 5 ml of expansion fluid. Spatulate vigorously and then place in a vacuum chamber to eliminate air from the mix.

6 Hold the duplicating flask on the vibrator with a low setting and feed the refractory material from a spatula into one corner of the mould (Fig. 83). Allow it to flow evenly from the corner progressively to all parts of the mould. Leave the refractory model to harden for 1 hour.

Partial dentures

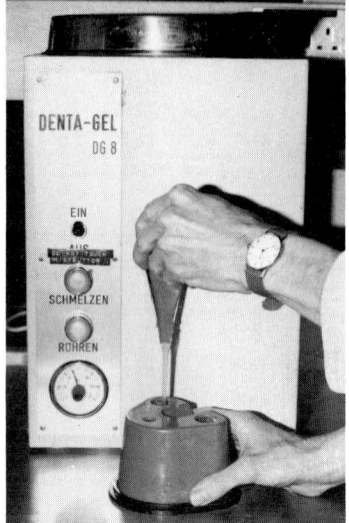

Fig. 80 Pouring duplicating gel from a thermostatically controlled bath.

Fig. 81 The base of the duplicating flask is removed and the gel cut from the cast to leave a bevel. The cast may then be levered from the gel with two wax knives.

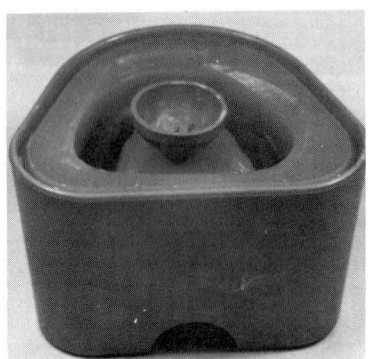

Fig. 82 The duplicating gel mould, with sprue former positioned, ready for the introduction of the investment material.

7 Carefully peel the duplicating medium from the cast and remove the sprue former (Fig. 84). Dry trim the refractory cast on a trimmer to fit an investing ring. Gently blow away any trimmings.

8 Place the investment in an oven at 93°C to dry out (Fig. 85). Whilst the cast is still warm, dip it into model hardener for 10 seconds. Leave to drain and warm again until any excess hardener has been absorbed. An hydrocal duplicate of the prepared master cast will also be required. This is the cast to which the metal frame will be fitted and on which the denture will be processed. Before pouring the gel mould for the hydrocal duplicate, remove the relief metal from the prepared master cast in the saddle regions. Use a powder/water ratio of 4:1 (200 g powder to 50 ml water) to prepare the hydrocal.

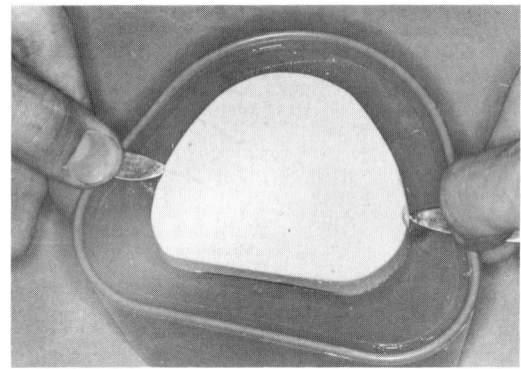

Preparing the wax pattern

In cold conditions, the wax pattern will adhere to the refractory cast more readily if the cast has been warmed slightly by the heat of an electric light bulb. Major components of the pattern are laid down first, finishing with the more detailed features.

1 Plate connectors, palatal bars and lingual bars are the first components to be laid down. A pointed India rubber or a small piece of sponge soaked in warm water and squeezed out is used to adapt a sheet of 0·45 mm casting wax to the cast (Fig. 86). Smooth out any folds which form in the wax. Where there is a high vaulted palate, either use 0·6 mm wax to avoid thinning the denture base at the height of the vault, or, using 0·45 mm wax, lay down the base pattern in right and left halves.

Laboratory procedures 2

2 Trim the wax to the required form of the plate or bar with a Le Cron carver. The inferior border of a lingual plate should be finished with a half pear-section wax rod.

3 Lay wax mesh over the relieved areas of the alveolar ridge in the edentulous spaces and seal the mesh to the pattern of the denture base. The mesh will form the bonding for the acrylic saddle when the denture is finally processed.

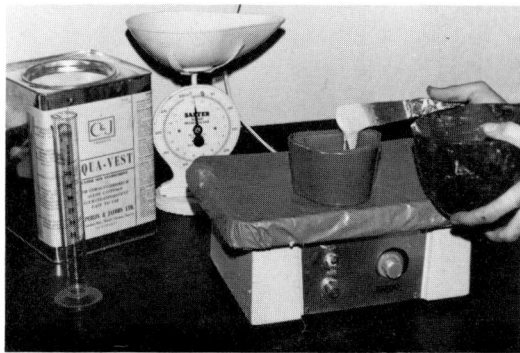

Fig. 83 The duplicating flask is placed on a vibrator and investment material introduced by small increments.

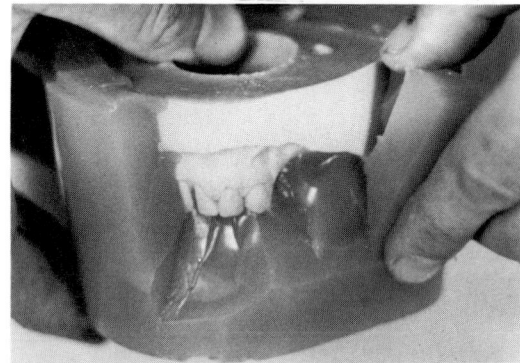

Fig. 84 The gel is removed from the flask and peeled from the set investment cast.

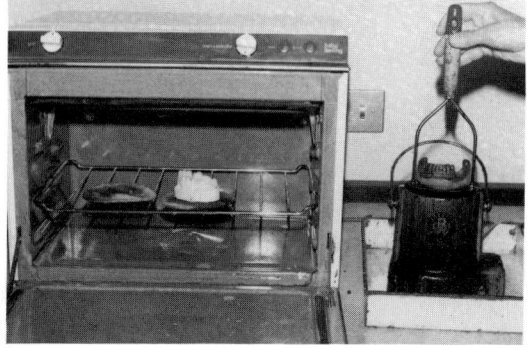

Fig. 85 The investment casts are dried in an oven at 93°C and dipped into a hardener.

Partial dentures

4 Lingual bars may be fashioned from half pear-shaped section wax rods. Similarly, clasp arms and connectors may be formed from suitable wax strands, tapered and thickened as required with inlay wax. Preformed wax patterns, i.e. for clasps, rests and connectors, are convenient aids for building up the overall pattern. These components should be accurately positioned and pressed firmly onto the investment cast.

5 The final details of the pattern, such as the heads of gingivally approaching clasps and occlusal rests are formed in inlay wax. Keep the occlusal rest patterns within the confine of the prepared seats. Wherever possible, finish the rests to a concave form, carving this with the spoon-shaped end of the Le Cron instrument. Rests formed in this manner are less bulky and will not interfere with the occlusion of the natural teeth: however, the rests must not be thinned to an extent where their rigidity is impaired.

6 Check that the wax pattern is completely sealed to the refractory cast: it is now ready for spruing.

Spruing

It is usually more convenient to sprue the pattern through the base of the refractory cast. Where there is complete palatal coverage, this arrangement will not be feasible and the pattern should be sprued to the posterior border. The number of sprues which are necessary is related to the efficiency of the casting machine to be used. Sprues should be kept to a minimum to reduce both the amount of metal to be melted and the trimming of the casting when complete. An

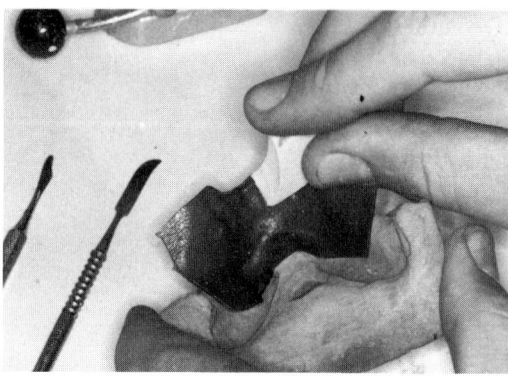

Fig. 86 Casting wax sheet may be adapted to the investment cast using a suitably shaped India rubber.

Laboratory procedures 2

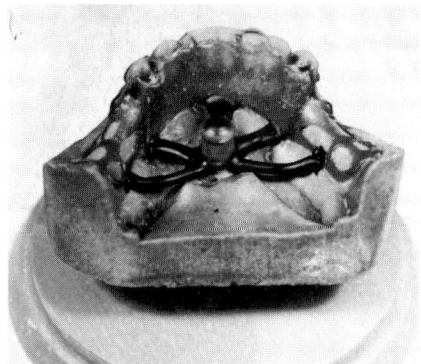

Fig. 87 The lower investment cast mounted and sprued through its base. The sprue former is beneath the cast.

efficient, modern induction machine will cast a metal framework through three sprues.

Spruing through the model base

1 Place the refractory cast on an investment ring base, with the cone former projecting through the hole in the base of the model (Fig. 87). Cement the cast to the base with sticky wax.

2 Use 2·5 mm diameter wax rod for the sprues. Run the sprues from the former to a thick region of the wax pattern (i.e. to a lingual plate or palatal bar, not to a clasp or mesh work). Position the sprues in such a manner that the molten metal will be able to flow into the final mould evenly and without turbulence.

Spruing from above

1 Mount the refractory cast on an investment ring base and lute in position with sticky wax (Fig. 88).

2 Place the refractory cast on the bench alongside the investment ring to be used.

3 The cone former is waxed to the posterior border of the plate connector and two subsidiary sprues are added either side of the former, which should stand 2–3 mm higher than the investment ring.

4 Ensure that the cone former is rigidly held and that the sprue position will allow the even flow of molten metal.

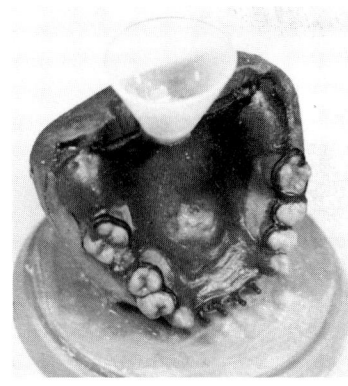

Fig. 88 The sprue former is waxed directly to the posterior border of the upper wax pattern with two auxiliary sprues extending laterally.

Partial dentures

Investing and casting the metal framework

1 With a soft brush, apply a coating of liquid investment to the wax pattern (Fig. 89).

2 Assemble the investing ring by fitting it to the rebate around the base. It is held in position by a clip applied to the everted flanges.

3 Prepare the investment by spatulating powder and water together in the ratio of 100 g to 14 ml. The actual amounts used will depend upon the size of the investment ring employed. Stand the mix under a vacuum bell to remove air bubbles.

4 Hold the investment ring on the vibrator operating at a low setting and introduce the investment using a spatula. The ring will thus fill from the base, the material flowing over the wax pattern. When the ring is full, remove it from the vibrator and allow to stand for 1 hour.

5 When the investment has set, unclip the ring to remove it. Hold the investment base down to remove the base plate and sprue former: in this way, fragments of investment will not fall back into the sprue hole.

6 Place the investment in a cold furnace and raise the temperature slowly with a low gas jet so that a temperature of 260°C AND NO MORE is achieved by the end of the first hour. This early slow heating is essential for the success of the casting.

7 After an hour, turn on the gas burners fully and heat the investment to 950°C over a second hour. Having achieved this temperature, allow the investment to heat soak for 20–30 minutes.

8 Prepare the induction casting machine for use employing the following sequences:

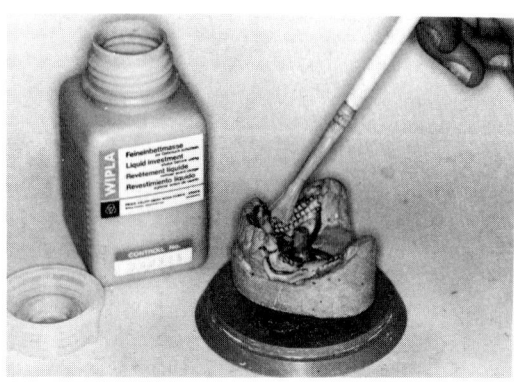

Fig. 89 Liquid investment is painted over the wax pattern before the cast is surrounded by the investment ring.

Laboratory procedures 2 **67**

a Switch on power, water (to cool the high frequency coil) and the argon gas (which provides an inert atmosphere over the metal in the crucible). An indicator light glows when the machine is ready for casting.
b Ensure the casting arm is correctly balanced for the size of casting ring to be employed.
c Select the heating stage for the amount of metal to be used:
Stage 1: up to 15 g metal.
Stage 2: 15–30 g metal.
Stage 3: more than 30 g metal.
9 Inspect the crucible and seat it in its mounting on the sliding mechanism.
10 Place the required amount of cobalt-chromium alloy in the crucible. 20 g is sufficient for an average denture.
11 Bring the casting ring from the furnace and place in position on the casting arm, aligning the sprue holes (Fig. 90, A, B).
12 Secure the sliding mechanism.
13 Position the observation glass above the crucible.

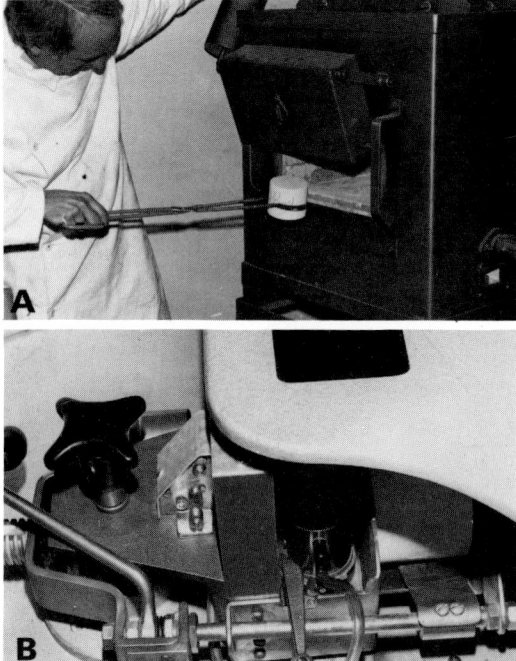

Fig. 90 (A) The investment mould being placed in a furnace. (B) The investment mould transferred to the craddle of the casting machine.

Partial dentures

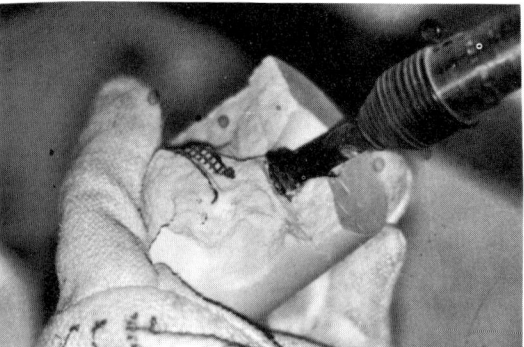

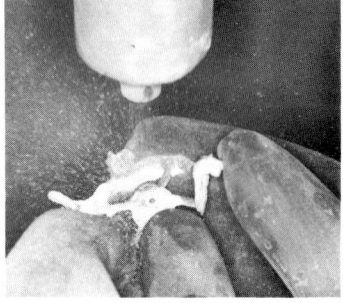

Fig. 91 The use of a pneumatic hammer in divesting a cobalt-chromium casting.

Fig. 92 Sandblasted castings cleaned of investment material.

14 Press the melting button and maintain it in the depressed position. Ensure that the ammeter reading does not exceed 1A.

15 Observe the melt through the glass and, when the ingots flow together, press the casting button. The motor will maintain the casting arm in motion for as long as the button is depressed. Casting time is of the order of 5 seconds and both melting and casting buttons should be held down for this period.

16 Allow the arm to come to rest of its own accord. Remove the casting ring to bench-cool for 20 minutes before plunging it in cold water.

Finishing the framework for insertion in the mouth

1 Use a pneumatic hammer to remove the remnants of investment from the casting (Fig. 91). In order to avoid damaging the more delicate framework, the hammer should be applied to the casting button. This procedure should be carried out in a divestment box in order to avoid scattering fragments of investment material.

2 Sandblast the casting to remove all remnants of investment and green oxide formations (Fig. 92).

3 Inspect the divested casting to ensure that it is complete. No porosity should be visible (Fig. 93).

4 Separate the sprues from the framework using cutting-off discs (Fig. 94). Remove the sprue stubs together with any surface blebs or flashes of cast metal with a tungsten carbide stone. Wear a visor to protect the eyes whilst undertaking this work or use a lathe where the cutting instrument is guarded by a protective screen (Fig. 95).

5 The metal framework is now fitted to the duplicate of the prepared master cast. Gently place the casting on the cast along the

Laboratory procedures 2

chosen path of insertion. Do not force the metal framework onto the cast, but observe any areas where the metal impinges upon it. Ease away the metal in these areas with an appropriately shaped stone. A successful denture framework should fit the cast accurately when seated: the only abrasion of the cast by the insertion of the framework should be of a very light nature at the tips of the clasps. If the cast is abraded in any other area, then the denture framework is unlikely to fit in the mouth.

6   The casting is now ready for electrobrightening, but before placing it in the bath, check that the electrolyte temperature has not been raised by constant earlier use. The optimum temperature is 18–20°C.

7   The denture framework is placed into an electrolyte bath 4–5 cm from an inert stainless steel cathode. A 12V current is supplied, either from a mains rectifier or battery, and the current flow is adjusted to 2A as registered on the ammeter (Fig. 96, A, B).

8   Leave the denture framework immersed in the polishing bath for

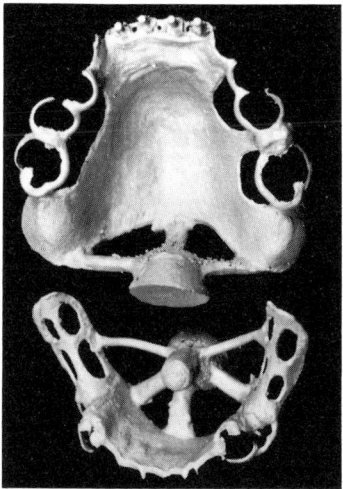

Fig. 93   When all traces of investment have been removed, the castings are ready for inspection.

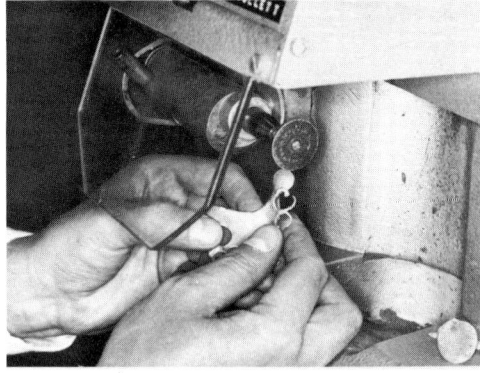

Fig. 94   Sprues are cut from the casting with a resin-bonded cutting-off disc.

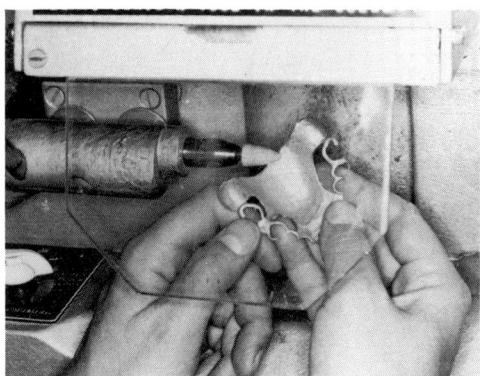

Fig. 95   The sprue stubs are trimmed down with a hard stone.

Partial dentures

5 minutes. Switch off the current, remove the framework and wash under running water. Lightly dry and replace the framework in the bath. Polish for a further 5 minutes. This method gives a superior result to immersing for 10 minutes without rinsing away the electrolytic debris.

9 Subsequent phases of polishing are undertaken by the mechanical abrasion of the metal surface by progressively finer agents. Careful waxing up and investment of the wax pattern minimises the time spent in the early stages of mechanical polishing, the first phase of which is the use of hard, impregnated rubber wheels and points (Fig. 97). These are mounted in a laboratory handpiece: the former are of special use in finishing the borders of the casting

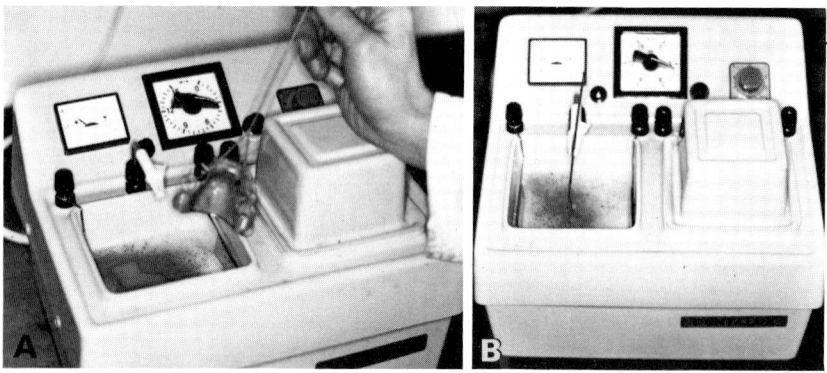

Fig. 96 (A) Inserting the casting into the electrolytic polishing bath. (B) The casting immersed in the bath. The electrolyte consists of 3 parts H_3PO_4, 1 part glycerine and 1 part water.

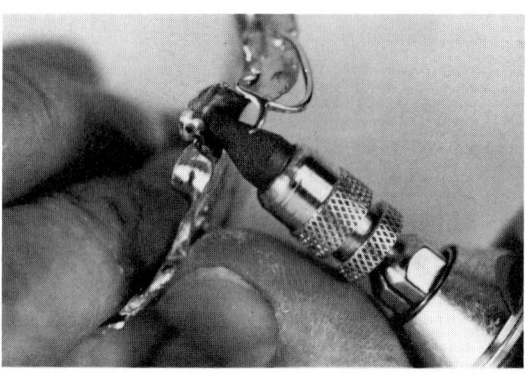

Fig. 97 A hard rubber point is useful for finishing clasps and the more detailed aspects of the metal framework.

Laboratory procedures 2

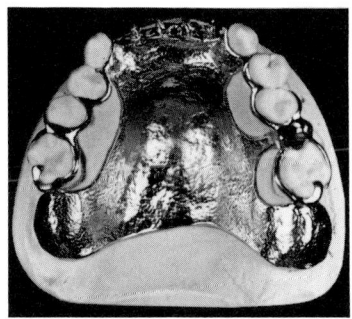

Fig. 98 The completed upper metal framework fitted to the master cast.

and the latter for polishing the more delicate components such as clasp arms.

10 To avoid the hazard of distorting the denture framework during polishing, it may be of advantage to set the casting in a plaster base which supports the fitting surface of the framework.

11 Polishing agents may be applied using a 5 cm diameter metal-centred hardbristle brush on a bench lathe or, for finer work, a hard felt disc mounted in a handpiece. Use the red polishing compound (which contains quartz-like particles) first and finish with the green compound (chrome oxide).

12 Remove the metal framework carefully from the plaster polishing block (if used) and clean off excess polishing agent with a denture brush and detergent. Rinse carefully.

13 Return the framework to the model and check that there has been no distortion during the polishing operation (Fig. 98).

Clinical stage 3

TRIAL INSERTION OF THE CAST FRAMEWORK

Objective

To ensure that the cast framework accurately fits the mouth and that no portion of the framework obstructs the occlusion of the natural teeth.

Instruments and materials (Fig. 99)

1. Mirror, probe and tweezers.
2. The metal framework mounted on duplicate cast.
3. Disclosing wax.
4. Typewriter correcting fluid.
5. Wax knife.
6. Articulating paper.
7. Laboratory handpiece and trimming stones.
8. Clean apron.
9. Clean headrest cover and square for bracket table.
10. Mouthwash and denture bowl.

Procedure

1 Place either the upper or the lower framework in the mouth and seat along the planned path of insertion. If difficulty is encountered, do not force the framework into position, but find the cause.

2 If necessary, gently warm a wax knife and apply a thin layer of disclosing wax to the fit surface of the framework where the discrepancy is suspected (Fig. 100, A, B). Even small errors in blocking out undercut regions parallel to the path of insertion may produce apparently gross errors of fit. Reinsert the framework and note the areas from which the wax has been displaced (Fig. 100, C). An alternative method of identifying areas in which a denture framework is bearing heavily is to use red stencil correcting fluid. This is supplied with a brush with which the fluid is painted on the fitting surfaces. The red dye is in a chloroform solvent which evaporates to leave the surface covered by the pigment. If seating of the framework is obstructed at any site, the red dye is rubbed away

Clinical stage 3

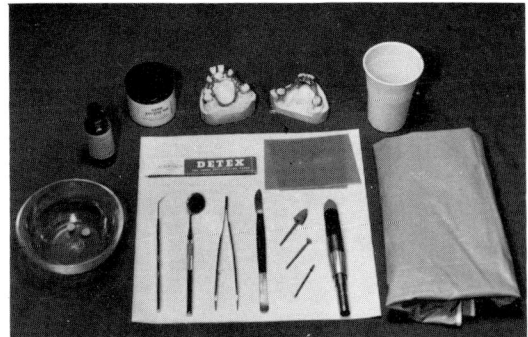

Fig. 99 The instruments and materials required for the trial insertion of the metal frameworks.

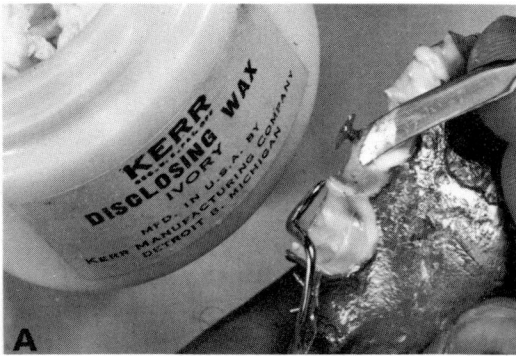

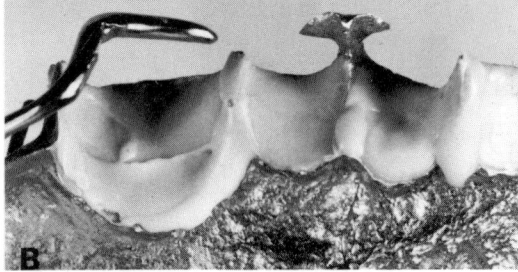

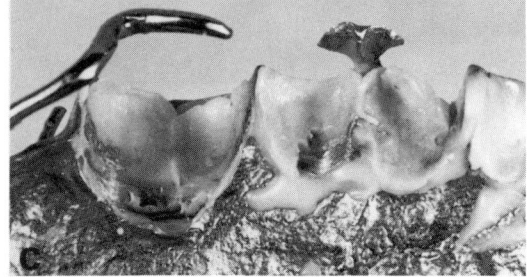

Fig. 100 (A) A thin layer of disclosing wax is flushed onto the area to be relieved from a warm Ash No. 5 instrument. (B) The completed application of disclosing wax ready for insertion into the mouth. (C) The wax has been displaced from areas of contact with tooth tissue on the fitting surface of two collets.

Partial dentures

leaving the metal exposed and indicating where adjustment is required.

3 Adjust the fit surface of the framework as indicated by the wax. Take care to avoid damage to the finishing edges of lingual plates which are occlusal to the survey lines, otherwise there will be a space between the denture and tooth surface resulting in food packing (Fig. 101). Dip the framework into a bowl of cold water from time to time to avoid overheating the framework and forming oxide deposits.

4 Wash away softened disclosing wax and metal trimmings: retry the framework in the mouth. Some improvement in fit should be noted, but the procedure may require repetition.

5 Should the metal framework show no early sign of an improvement in fit, then the more likely explanation of the situation lies in the probable distortion of the original impression: a new one will be required.

6 The denture framework should fit as well in the mouth as it does on a cast. Check the fit of the occlusal rests with a probe (Fig. 102). Use a mouth mirror to ensure that the upper base plate or palatal connectors are in close apposition to the palatal mucosa.

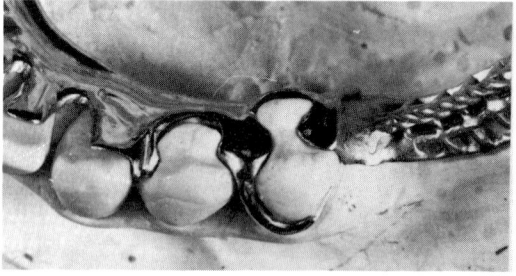

Fig. 101 The framework has been carelessly eased on the lingual aspect of the two premolar teeth. As a result, contact between the teeth and the lingual plate connector has been lost to produce a food packing hazard.

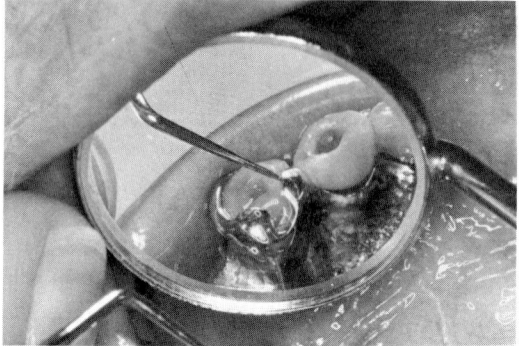

Fig. 102 The fit of the occlusal rests is checked using a mouth mirror and probe.

Clinical stage 3 75

7 With a single framework in the mouth, check the patient's occlusion. Occlusal contacts of the natural teeth should not be hindered by the framework. If the occlusal contacts are not as planned, locate the obstruction by the framework with articulating paper and correct.

8 Remove the framework when correctly fitted and repeat the procedure with the second framework.

9 Finally, check the patient's occlusion with both frameworks in the mouth to ensure that there is no metal to metal occlusal obstruction. At this stage we should consider the special problems of support presented by particular clinical situations as these may necessitate additional clinical and laboratory procedures.

SPECIAL PROBLEMS OF THE DISTAL EXTENSION SADDLE

We have seen that when the support of different saddles varies between rigid tooth support and displaceable mucus membrane, movement of the denture framework may take place. In the case of the distal extension saddle illustrated (Fig. 103, A–D), tooth support is provided by the rest on the mesial abutment. This results in pressure being concentrated on the mucoperiosteum at the distal end, whereas that adjacent to the abutment tooth bears no load at all. When the denture is being retained by an occlusally approaching clasp, which encircles the abutment tooth, leverage is applied to the tooth which stresses the periodontal membrane. The use of a gingivally approaching clasp may protect the abutment from this damaging stress but nevertheless the load on the alveolus remains concentrated at the distal end of the saddle. Such a concentration of load on a small area of mucoperiosteum is likely to accelerate bone resorption and allow the saddle to sink out of occlusion.

The purpose of 'stress breaking' is to protect the abutment teeth from harmful leverage and to allow the supporting mucoperiosteum and bone to be uniformly loaded. It involves the incorporation of a flexible component between the rigid retainer element and the mucosal-borne saddle. Examples of stress breaking designs are illustrated in Fig. 104, A–G. The difficulty is to allow the base to move under the influence of occlusal load according to the displaceability of the supporting mucus membrane. One way which has been advocated for relieving the stress on the abutment tooth is the hinged attachment, which allows the distal extension base to rotate. This does not allow the supporting tissues to

Partial dentures

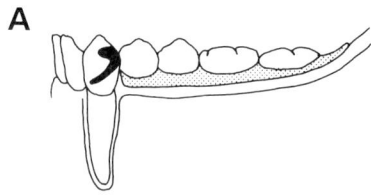

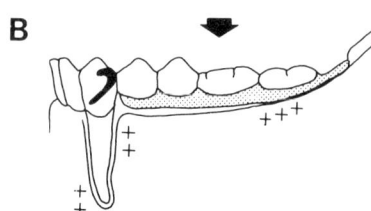

Fig. 103 (A) A distal extension saddle denture with encircling clasps and rests upon the abutment teeth. The denture has been made on a cast obtained from a mucostatic impression. (B) The same mouth when an occlusal load is applied. Note that pressure is concentrated on the mucosa at the distal end of the saddle and leverage is being applied to the abutment tooth. (C) By using a bar clasp, the damaging stress upon the abutment teeth is reduced but the load is still concentrated on a small area of mucoperiosteum. (D) By means of the Applegate fluid wax technique the mucoperiosteum supporting the saddle has been displaced so that, under functional loads, the displacement of the mucoperiosteum is similar to that of the periodontal membrane supporting the abutment teeth.

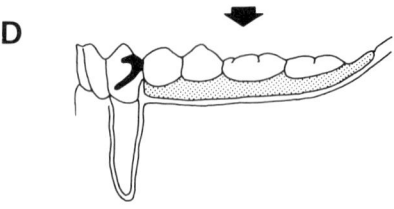

be evenly loaded and lateral stresses will still be transmitted to the framework of the denture and thus to the teeth. A long lingual bar connector attached to the framework in the lingual sulcus in the midline is another attempt at 'stress breaking'. Since this allows movement to take place about a wider arc the mucoperiosteum is more evenly loaded. Connectors of this type are poorly tolerated by the tongue and the movement which takes place at the point of union of the flexible and more rigid elements attracts a salivary film by capillary action. This results in plaque developing which causes

Clinical stage 3

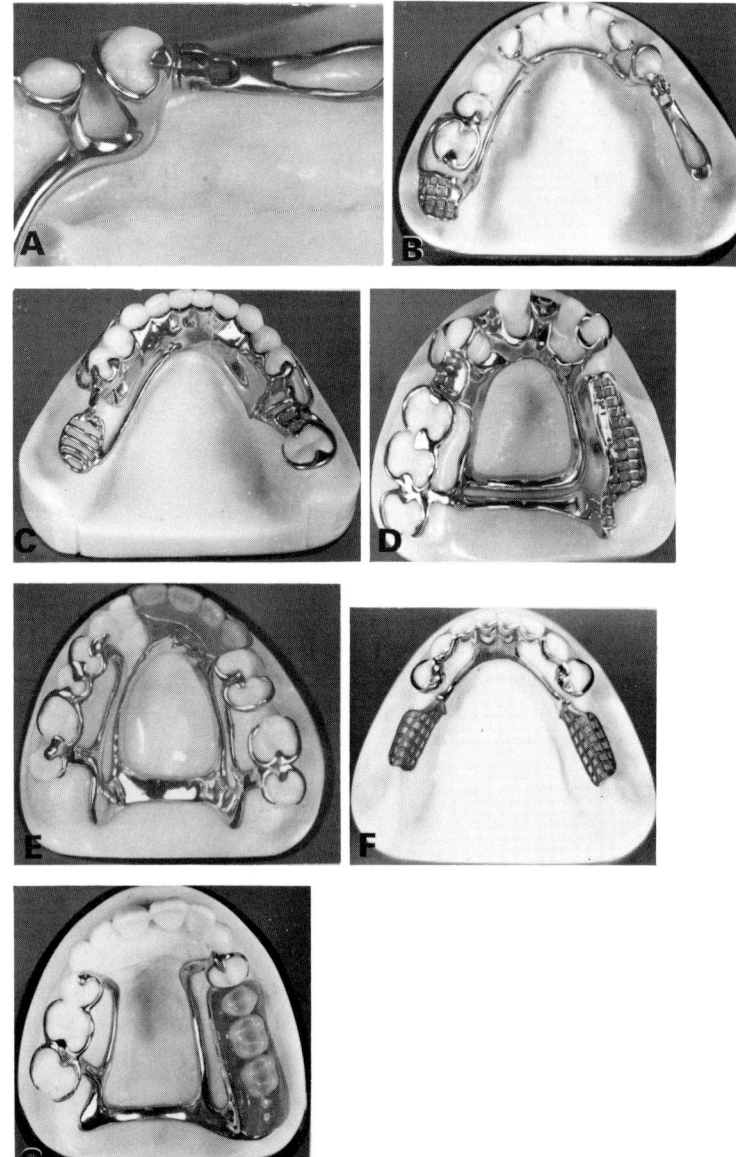

Fig. 104 (A, B) Examples of hinged distal extension saddles. (C–G) Denture frameworks in which saddles are attached by flexible connectors: these connectors are designed to act in a 'stress breaking' fashion.

Partial dentures

inflammation of the adjacent soft tissues which may then be traumatised by the moving elements.

A further problem with this type of stress breaker arises because the elements of the denture base adjacent to the abutment tooth may compress the gingival margin distal to that tooth. Whilst the principles of stress breaking are usually illustrated by means of the use of a distal extension saddle, it may be applied in any situation where support is obtained partially from natural teeth and partially from the yielding mucoperiosteum. The upper anterior bounded saddle is an example where compensation often needs to be provided for the differences in the nature of the support tissues. If an entirely rigid metal framework is provided in this situation, pressure applied at the front of the mouth will result in movement of the base resting on the displaceable tissue and the resultant leverage will cause the retainers on the posterior teeth to be forced out of the retentive undercuts. This may be avoided if tooth support can be provided at each end of the saddle, but the abutment teeth (usually canines) need to be prepared with rest seats which can effectively oppose the vertical movement taking place. A rest placed on the inclined palatal surface of the canine will not prevent movement.

The alternative to stress breaking is to so reduce the movement of the saddle that the abutment teeth are not damaged. Therefore the support from the teeth and the mucoperiosteum beneath the distal extension saddles must be equilibrated. This is the purpose of the tissue displacement impression technique described by Applegate. The procedure necessitates an additional appointment and an acrylic tray or trays will first need to be added to the denture framework.

Laboratory procedures 3(a)

Adding acrylic tray to the distal extension framework

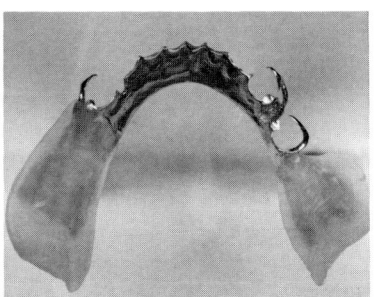

Fig. 105 Acrylic trays added to the lower denture framework.

Outline the limits of the distal extension saddle with a pencil and lay down a 0·25 mm thickness of casting wax to cover the saddle area. This will provide a space beneath the acrylic tray to accommodate the impression wax. When the wax spacer has hardened, dust with French chalk. Now seat the denture framework into place on the cast. Ensure that there is sufficient clearance around the framework for the attachment of the resin tray material. Prepare a sheet of self curing acrylic and adapt it to the retentive framework, covering the whole of the saddle area with a sufficient thickness of material to produce a rigid tray. After hardening of the resin, the framework is removed from the cast and the tray is trimmed to remove any excess material (Fig. 105).

Clinical stage 3(a)

DESCRIPTION OF THE FLUID WAX TECHNIQUE FOR RECORDING AN IMPRESSION OF DISTAL EXTENSION SADDLE AREAS

Instruments and materials (Fig. 106)

1. Water bath with thermostatic control.
2. Camel hair artists' brush.
3. Impression wax.
4. Low fusing compound.
5. Plastikarver acrylic trimmer.
6. Handpiece.

Objective

To protect the abutment tooth from damaging forces by recording an impression of the mucoperiosteum supporting the distal extention saddle under a controlled displacing force.

Procedure

Try-in the metal framework with the acrylic tray attachment and check the extension. If the flanges are overextended, trim these with the acrylic trimmer. Ensure that the mylohyoid muscle is adequately

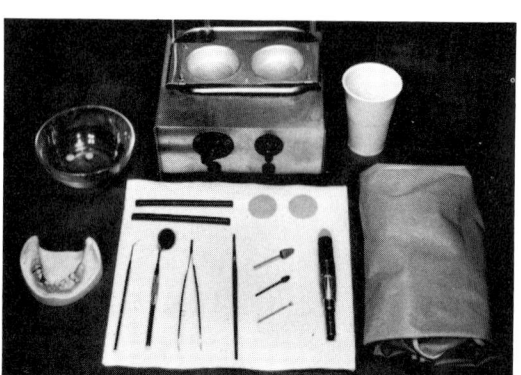

Fig. 106 Instruments and materials for recording the wax displacement impression.

Clinical stage 3(a)

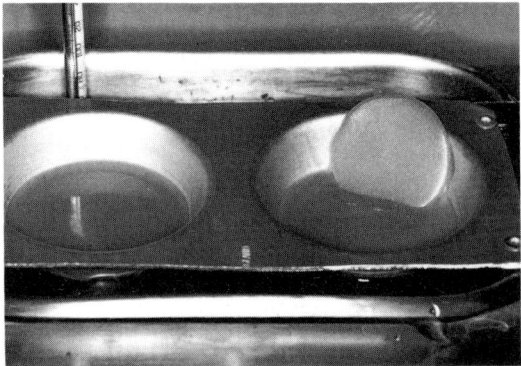

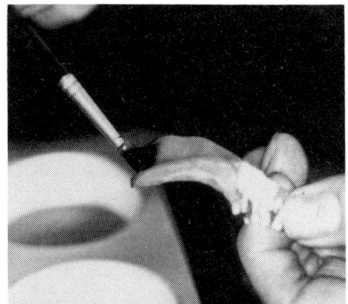

Fig. 107 Impression wax is melted over a water bath.

Fig. 108 The fluid wax is painted onto the fit surface of the tray with a brush.

relieved. If the border of the tray does not reach the full sulcus depth, apply softened low fusing compound to the border, flame, temper and reseat the framework. Direct the patient to make muscular movements which will ensure moulding of the compound. When the extension of the tray is correct, slightly relieve the tissue surface of the compound by scraping with a sharp knife. Ensure that there are no undercut areas on the fitting surface of the tray, which might cause the impression wax to be dragged, and the tray is now ready for the application of the wax.

Applegate suggested a wax impression technique for distal extension saddles and developed the wax for this purpose. Unfortunately, the manufacturer who produced the material has now ceased to do so. McCrorie (1982) devised a recipe* for a material, with suitable flow properties at mouth temperature, which could be made up from other available waxes. This produces a controlled displacement of the mucoperiosteum which is sufficient to stabilise the denture, yet insufficient to occlude the capillaries and cause tissue morbidity.

A disc of wax is allowed to melt in a metal cup suspended in a water bath (Fig. 107) and the thermostat set to provide a water temperature of 67°C. Dry the surface of the acrylic. Dip the brush into the molten wax and paint the tissue surface of the saddle with an even layer of wax (Fig. 108). Carefully reposition the framework in the mouth pressing the occlusal rests down onto their seatings (Fig. 109). (NOTE: No pressure should be applied to the saddle itself. The

---

* McCrorie's recipe: 25% yellow beeswax (BDH Chemicals), 75% paraffin wax (Thermowax, R.A. Lamb, London NW10), colouring (Candle Makers Supplies, London W14).

Partial dentures

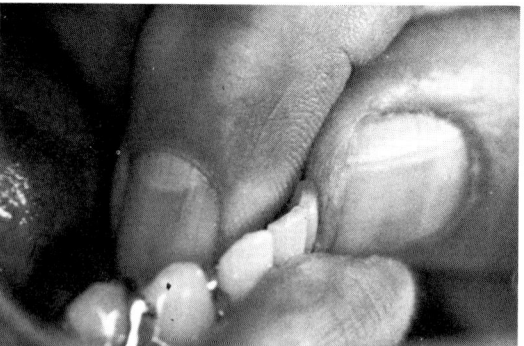

Fig. 109 The framework is returned to the mouth and held in position by finger pressure applied to the major connector.

viscosity of the wax at mouth temperature displaces the underlying soft tissues; pressure in excess of this may cause occlusion of the vessels supplying the mucous membrane, with subsequent atrophy of the tissue.)

Hold the framework firmly in position for one minute to allow the wax to flow and then request the patient to make functional movements to mould the periphery. The impression is then removed and inspected (Fig. 110). Where the wax is in firm contact with the mucosa under a supporting load, the surface will be glossy. Where the shiny surface has not been developed, it will be necessary to brush on more molten wax and to reseat the framework until an even glossy surface is obtained. Before each addition of wax, the impression surface must be completely dried under a gentle stream of compressed air. If the tray is inadequately relieved, the wax should be removed from the site. The base is trimmed to provide liberal relief and the procedure is repeated. When excess wax is added to the acrylic tray it will resist the seating of the metal framework. Sufficient time must be allowed for the surplus wax to flow, otherwise the rests will not fit on the occlusal surface of the abutment teeth. This is the commonest cause of error in the application of this technique. To ensure that it does not occur the framework must be held in position for 10 minutes after the initial even gloss has been obtained.

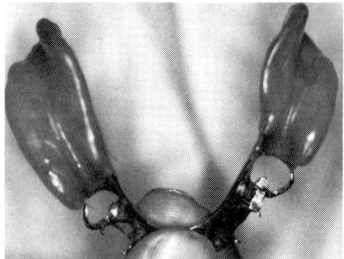

Fig. 110 The completed wax impression. Note the smooth gloss finish and rolled borders.

Laboratory procedures 3(b)

Altering the cast by means of the fluid wax impression

The edentulous distal extension of the original cast represents the supporting tissues recorded with a mucostatic impression material. The wax impression has consolidated these tissues under the displacing effect of the wax and the cast must now be modified to

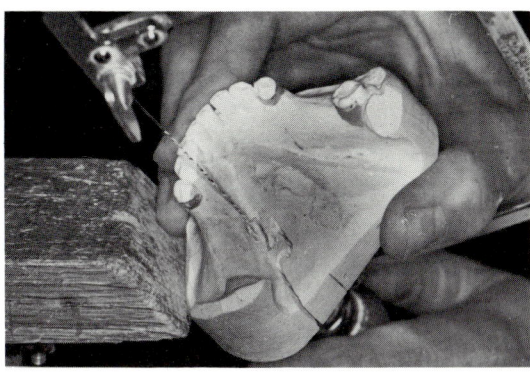

Fig. 111 The saddle is cut from the cast with a fretsaw.

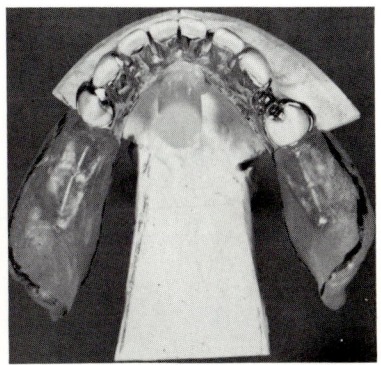

Fig. 112 A bilateral distal extension cast prepared for modification. The denture frame has been repositioned in readiness for the new sections to be poured.

represent the altered conditions of loading. The original cast is sectioned at the distal surface of the last abutment tooth/teeth (Fig. 111) and the portion representing the distal support is removed (Fig. 112). The framework bearing the fluid wax impression is now seated on the supporting teeth and, with the cast inverted, a stone slurry is vibrated into place in the wax impression. The reconstituted cast is trimmed and the trays removed from the framework. Wax bases are attached to the denture frameworks in saddle areas, to which wax rims are added.

Clinical stage 4

JAW RELATIONSHIPS

Objective

To record the definitive jaw relationships and to select replacement teeth.

Instruments and materials

1. Denture frameworks (with wax rims) mounted on the master casts.
2. Mirror, probe and tweezers.
3. Modelling wax.
4. Wax knife.
5. Clean apron.
6. Clean headrest cover and a square for the bracket table.
7. Mouthwash and denture bowl.

Procedure

The procedure adopted for the registration of the definitive jaw relationship is identical to that followed when establishing a relationship for the study casts (see pp. 16 et seq.). The only difference is that the rims are mounted on the denture frameworks and not on self-cure acrylic bases. It can be appreciated why such emphasis has been laid on ensuring that occlusal rests and clasp connectors do not interfere with the occlusion at the trial insertion of the denture frameworks: a true relationship cannot be registered in the presence of such interferences. There are two reasons for reregistering the jaw relationship at this stage. They are related to the differences between the study casts and master casts in respect of the occlusal preparation and, perhaps, the alteration of a cast following a wax displacement impression. When anterior teeth are to be replaced, the rim is adjusted to provide the correct lip support and horizontal and vertical overlap with the opposing incisor teeth. The centre line should also be marked to provide a complete prescription for the setting of the replacement teeth.

When the relationship has been recorded, transfer the denture frameworks and rims to the master casts. Check that the casts may be accurately located in the relationship recorded. If there is any doubt, then the cuspal registration in the wax rims should be improved. Confirm that the heels of the casts are not contacting and preventing the teeth from coming together in their correct occlusal relationship. When satisfied with the registration, the facebow record is obtained (see p. 16).

Selection of teeth

Although the presence of natural teeth may provide the operator with particulars of the shape and mould of teeth required to restore the edentulous space, matching of the teeth may prove to be difficult. One manufacturer may make a tooth of the correct shade but with inappropriate moulds, or the reverse may be true. Teeth which appear to match the natural abutments when the framework is absent may have an unsatisfactory appearance when supported by a metal backing. Several different shade and mould guides may need to be consulted before suitable teeth are found and modifications of the mould may be needed to produce a tooth of pleasing appearance. Acrylic teeth are most commonly used on partial dentures due to limitations in space. Whereas these teeth may be ground to fit into the space available the necessary grinding of porcelain teeth might eliminate the diatoric holes used for anchorage and so weaken the tooth as to render it liable to fracture. When isolated teeth are to be replaced the teeth may be fitted directly to the ridge without any acrylic flange. The cast should be scraped to a depth of $\frac{1}{2}$ mm and the tooth carefully ground to fit closely to the cast. Whereas this procedure results in a pleasing appearance of the tooth fitted to the gum it may not be practicable if, through prolonged absence of the tooth to be replaced, the alveolar process has resorbed to leave a depression in this situation. In such a case it becomes necessary to add gumwork to restore the labial contour. Such isolated additions of gumwork need to be carefully blended with the alveolar process.

When selecting posterior teeth, moulds should be selected of narrow buccolingual width. Premolars should be of sufficient length as they are often seen when the patient smiles and a short artificial premolar tooth set adjacent to a long canine gives an unnatural appearance. The mesiodistal dimension will be dictated by the space which is available.

Laboratory procedures 4

Setting the teeth for trial insertion

The selected teeth should be set in wax attached to the denture framework which is positioned on the modified master cast on the articulator. Their position will be determined by the need to establish a satisfactory occlusion with opposing natural or artificial teeth, to achieve a degree of balanced articulation (in bilateral distal extension cases) and to meet cosmetic requirements. After they have been suitably arranged, wax should be built up to represent gumwork where required and carefully carved to simulate the natural contour of the alveolar process and gingival margins.

Clinical stage 5

TRIAL INSERTION

Objectives

1 To check that the teeth are arranged correctly in the arch and that they occlude satisfactorily.
2 To ensure that the appearance of the trial denture is satisfactory.

Instruments and materials for trial insertion

1 Denture frameworks mounted on the articulator with teeth waxed into position.
2 Mirror, probe and tweezers.
3 Modelling wax.
4 Wax knife.
5 Clean apron.
6 Clean headrest cover and a square for the bracket table.
7 Mouthwash and denture bowl.

Procedure

The framework with the teeth waxed into position must now be tried in the patient's mouth. As the framework has already been checked and the teeth have been waxed into position on a cast from which all unwanted undercuts have been removed, the dentures should be positioned without impediment. The occlusion is checked to ensure even contact at the desired level and if any discrepancy is observed, a new occlusal registration may need to be recorded. This will necessitate removing the teeth, replacing them with wax upon which the new recordings are made. Assuming that the trial dentures are satisfactory, the patient should be given a mirror and invited to comment upon the appearance of the dentures. Every effort should be made to meet the patient's reasonable requests, but sometimes patients will object to the presence of extra-coronal retainers on canines and premolars. It must be explained to them that they have an important part to play in the successful functioning of the prosthesis and have been placed in the least obtrusive positions. (Some discussion should have taken place with the patient at an earlier stage concerning the need for this component.)

Laboratory procedures 5

PROCESSING THE DENTURE

The wax in which the teeth have been set and which represents the mucosal tissue must now be replaced with acrylic resin. The waxed up denture is seated on the duplicate master cast, and the edges of the wax are sealed to the underlying cast so that the investing plaster or stone cannot run beneath the denture. The cast is then embedded in plaster in the deeper part of the flask. It may be necessary to reduce the base of the cast to enable it to be lowered into the flask. The plaster should cover all the metal framework, clasps and rests, and only the replacement teeth should be exposed with their supporting wax in a gentle hollow in the surface of the plaster (Fig. 113). When the plaster has set and dried, it is painted with an alginate separating solution which penetrates into the surface of the plaster and covers it with a thin protective skin. The other section of the flask is filled with a 50:50 plaster/artificial stone mix which is also vibrated into place over the surface of the teeth and wax, before the two sections of the flasks are brought together and closed by pressure in the bench press. Set the flask aside for one hour to allow the plaster/stone mix to set, and then immerse it in boiling water for 10 minutes to soften the wax, so facilitating the parting of the two sections of the flask. Remove the softened wax remaining in the flask and wash the moulds with boiling water. This will remove any wax remaining.

It is particularly important that no wax residue is left on the surface of the teeth as this would interfere with the anchorage of the teeth to the denture base resin. The flasked moulds should be allowed to stand overnight before packing. This will allow the plaster to reach its full strength and will ensure that the mould is

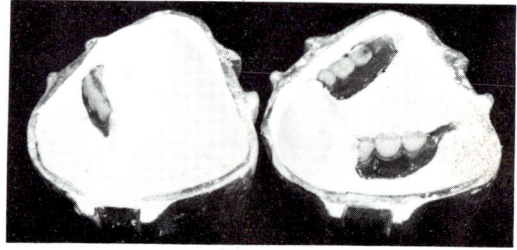

Fig. 113 The upper and lower dentures have been invested in the deeper sections of their respective flasks. Only the replacement teeth and supporting wax are exposed.

Laboratory procedures 5

completely cooled. Examine the margins of the gypsum moulds for thin edges which could fracture during packing: these should be trimmed. A separating medium is now applied to the plaster surfaces, taking care once more that none runs onto the surface of the teeth. After the separating medium has been allowed to dry, the mould should be packed with acrylic dough, which is covered with a sheet of damp cellophane to prevent the resin adhering to the investing gypsum during a trial closure. The flask pressure should be slowly raised to avoid fracturing any of the investing plaster. On opening the flask, any surplus resin which has been extruded is removed. If no surplus resin is present, a little more dough should be added and a further trial closure should be carried out. After this the cellophane is removed, the flask is finally closed and processing effected in the normal manner. After processing the denture is removed from the flask, trimmed and polished (Fig. 114). It is then placed back on the master cast. Should the blocking out of undercuts have been incorrect it will be necessary to trim the acrylic, before the denture will fit the cast. Should there have been any error in processing which affects the vertical dimension of the denture the resulting occlusal discrepancy may be removed by grinding on the articulator.

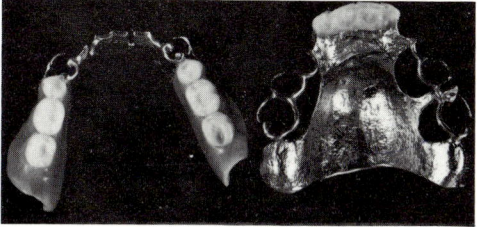

Fig. 114 The completed dentures ready for insertion.

Clinical stage 6

FITTING THE COMPLETED DENTURES

Objectives

1 To check the fit, occlusion and retention of the completed dentures.
2 To instruct the patient in the correct use of the denture and of the importance of good oral hygiene measures.

Instruments and materials (Fig. 115)

1 Mirror, probe and tweezers.
2 Completed denture.
3 Articulating paper.
4 Disclosing wax.
5 Wax knife.
6 Wax wafer and water bath.
7 Laboratory handpiece and trimmer.
8 Clean apron.
9 Clean headrest cover and square for bracket table.
10 Mouthwash and denture bowl.

Procedure

As the completed denture has already been fitted to the master cast, no further adjustment should be necessary to seat it in the mouth. If

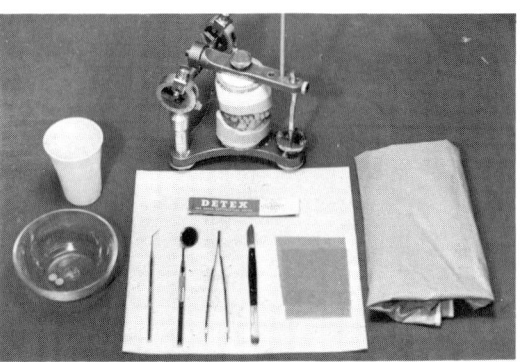

Fig. 115 Instruments and materials required when fitting the completed dentures.

it fails to go into place there has been an error in the blocking out of undercuts and the master cast will have been abraded as the denture has been forced onto it. Careful examination of the cast will reveal where the denture should be eased.

If the denture seats down on the cast but there are discrepancies in the occlusion when the articulator is closed, this will be due to changes which have taken place during processing of the acrylic. If there was an error in the original jaw relationship record, this will not be apparent when the case is seated on the articulator and will only be manifest when the denture is seated in the mouth. If the denture is wholly supported by the teeth, it may be possible to correct this error by identifying the discrepancy in the mouth with articulating paper. But, if the denture is partly supported by the mucoperiosteum, it is wise to record a precontact registration of centric relation and thus identify any premature contacts by remounting the case on the articulator. In both circumstances the teeth are carefully ground to establish the optimum occlusal relationship.

Plaster of Paris is the medium preferred for registering the precontact centric relation. However, in a partially edentulous case, there is danger that the liquid plaster may flow and engage undercuts in natural teeth. For this reason a specially manufactured 'wafer' is used. The wax, which has metallic filings incorporated in it to ensure good heat conduction, is heated in a water bath to produce even softening of the wax facilitating an accurate jaw relation record.

The dentures will have been designed about a planned path of insertion and withdrawal and the patient should be shown how to insert and remove each denture without excessive force or stress being applied to the denture or abutment teeth. Care must be taken to ensure that the mucous membrane of the cheek is not trapped between clasp arm and tooth as the denture is seated.

DENTURE AND ORAL HYGIENE

It should be explained to the patient that the wearing of a denture will increase susceptibility to caries and periodontal disease. The denture will have been designed to minimise this risk but a high standard of denture and oral hygiene is important. Partial dentures should be removed from the mouth after each meal and cleaned with a moistened toothbrush to remove loose adherent particles. The use of toothpaste relying upon a mild abrasive action for cleaning should be discouraged as over a long period of time this may be damaging to the denture base resin. The patient should also clean the natural teeth

Partial dentures

after each meal to remove debris which may accumulate in sites protected from the cleansing action of the tongue. Because the wearing of dentures increases the likelihood of plaque retention on the natural teeth he should be shown how to reveal it with disclosing tablets. At night, the denture should be removed and stored in an aqueous medium and it is convenient to use a denture cleansing solution. Where metal components have been incorporated in the denture, it is wise to avoid solutions of hypochlorites but rather to use the oxygen-liberating alkaline perborate or percarbonate-based cleansers. Before returning the dentures to the mouth, they should be carefully rinsed to remove any of the chemical cleanser. Because of the complexity of the denture, patients sometimes experience difficulty in cleaning the inside of clasps. A simple means of doing this is to tie a piece of cord to the washtap and to gently strop the fitting surface of the denture against it. This effectively removes plaque and keeps the surface of the denture polished (Fig. 116).

The patient should be encouraged to handle the dentures with great care for, although they have been designed to withstand stresses generated in the mouth, they may easily be damaged if dropped on hard surfaces. It is for this reason that brushing or stropping should be carried out over a basin full of water which will cushion them against an accidental fall.

INSTRUCTIONS CONCERNING USE OF THE DENTURES

The patient should be told not to expect immediate restoration of full efficiency with partial dentures. Indeed, if there are many teeth lost and the partial denture is partly or wholly mucosal-borne, then he

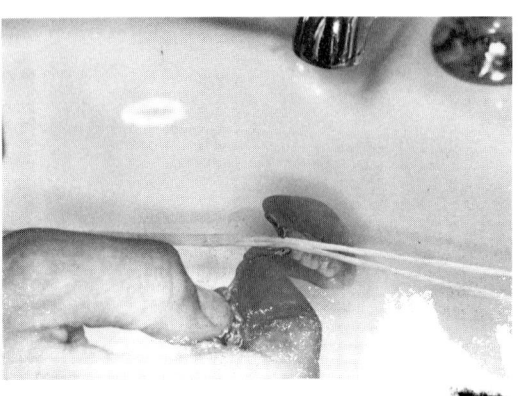

Fig. 116 The use of floss to clean the fitting surface of a clasp.

need expect the limitations similar to those imposed by complete dentures. During the first weeks after receiving the denture the diet should be restricted so that items requiring considerable masticatory force are avoided. Food should be cut into small pieces before being placed in the mouth. Should the tissues supporting the denture become sore or inflamed, the denture should be left out but it should be replaced 24 hours before the next visit so that the inflamed area can be easily identified and adjustment made to the denture. A patient should never be told to persevere. If the mouth is hurting then something is likely to be wrong and this must be diagnosed and treated. Very occasionally the tolerance of the supporting tissues is so low that dentures cannot be worn. There may be a psychological reason for the dentures being rejected by the patient, and if either of these possibilities exist the case should be referred for a consultant opinion.

Clinical stage 7

ADJUSTMENT OF THE DENTURE

Objectives

To identify and correct any errors of occlusion or of fit which may have caused the patient discomfort.

Instruments and materials (Fig. 117)

1   Mirror, probe and tweezers.
2   Modelling wax.
3   Wax knife.
4   Clean apron.
5   Clean headrest cover and square for bracket table.
6   Mouthwash and denture bowl.

Procedure

The patient should be given an appointment to return within 1 week so that it may be ascertained whether the dentures are causing any discomfort. The mouth should be examined for any signs of injury.

If the denture is entirely supported by the abutment teeth, discomfort will be due either to excessive pressure being applied to a tooth or impingement of the denture on the edentulous ridge or gingivae. A tight fit of the metal framework should have been

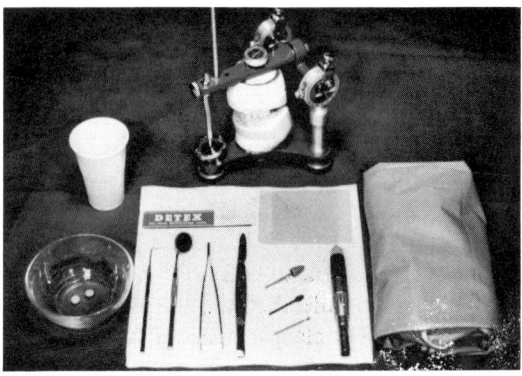

Fig. 117 Instruments and materials necessary for adjusting the dentures.

Clinical stage 7

revealed and corrected at the trial insertion stage but if it was overlooked a disclosing medium should be used to identify the area requiring to be eased. If the occlusion should be heavy on an occlusal rest, this would have the effect of producing 'wedging' between teeth and the faulty occlusal relationship should be identified and corrected. Pressure on the gingivae or alveolar mucosa must be identified by the use of disclosing wax and corrected by grinding. Remember that an inflamed mucosa will be swollen and when the irritant is removed it will become reduced in size.

If the denture is wholly or partially supported by the mucoperiosteum, soreness may be due to excess pressure being brought about by an error in jaw relationship. Before relieving the denture over any sore area, therefore, the occlusion of the teeth should be checked and any premature contacts or obstruction to free movement identified. Such errors should be corrected after remounting the casts on an articulator by means of a check record. Only after it has been ensured that the occlusal relationships are correct should pressure areas beneath the denture be identified with disclosing wax. If it has been necessary to adjust the denture the patient should be invited to return for a further examination one week later.

Review of dentures in service

The patient should be recommended to return for dental inspection at six-monthly intervals, when the teeth and their supporting tissues should be examined for the presence of caries and periodontal disease. On these occasions the partial dentures should be checked to see that they are functioning satisfactorily and have not suffered any deterioration through mishandling by the patient.

Damage to partial dentures can occur during insertion and removal and by inappropriate handling during cleaning. Attention should be paid to the fit of the denture and in particular to the clasps on the abutment teeth. If a clasp no longer makes contact with the surface of a tooth, it may be possible to adjust it. Care must be taken to see that the clasp is not engaging too deep an undercut. This is the most common cause of a deformed clasp as the elastic limit of the material is exceeded when the clasp is removed from its undercut. If it is not possible to adjust the clasp and it is adjacent to an acrylic saddle, then the clasp should be replaced by one of improved design. The clasp is removed from the denture which is then positioned in the mouth so that an impression of the arch may be obtained with the denture *in situ*. The impression is withdrawn containing the partial denture and it is then a straightforward matter to pour a new cast on which the denture is already mounted. The abutment tooth is surveyed and the appropriate positioning for the new clasp tip is determined with the aid of an undercut gauge. The connector for the new clasp is embedded in the acrylic saddle.

If resorption of edentulous alveolar processes has occurred the denture will sink in those areas supported by the mucoperiosteum. This not only results in the loss of contact with the occlusal surface of the teeth in the opposing jaw, but could result in stress being transmitted to the abutment tooth. Rebasing of saddles which have undergone resorption is essential in preserving function. The use of the fluid wax technique described in Clinical stage 3A may be adopted for this purpose. It is important to remember that after the dentures have been rebased the occlusion is also checked to ensure that any resultant imperfection is corrected.

Appendix

ACRYLIC PARTIAL DENTURES

Indications

Although a metal framework is desirable for most partial dentures because the strength which the metal imparts permits a more hygienic design, a partial denture with an all-acrylic base may be prescribed in any of the following circumstances:

1 To prevent drifting of teeth following the premature loss of an anterior tooth from a young patient's mouth.
2 As a rapid and temporary replacement of an anterior tooth extracted from an adult's mouth.
3 Where there is deemed to be inadequate support potential from the remaining natural teeth for a tooth-borne denture.
4 Where it can be foreseen that a tooth of poor prognosis may require extraction and a replacement added to the denture in coming months.
5 When the patient is to receive complete immediate insertion dentures without previous denture-wearing experience and a training or treatment denture is deemed advisable.

Procedure for construction

The stages in the construction of an acrylic-based partial denture are similar to those for a metal denture.

Clinical work

>Primary impressions.
>Secondary impressions.
>Jaw relations.
>Trial insertion.
>Insertion and check record.

Laboratory work

>Study casts.
>Occlusion rims.
>Set up teeth.
>Process denture.

Partial dentures

These stages may be modified in the production of the more simple denture, for example, where a temporary one-tooth denture is to be made for an otherwise intact arch. In such an instance, one set of impressions is adequate and the denture may be fitted at the subsequent visit.

Design

A form of acrylic denture commonly found consists of a base which fits around the lingual surfaces of the remaining natural teeth in a series of collets and is devoid of clasps. These devices prise the teeth apart slightly as they are inserted and may be heard to 'click' into

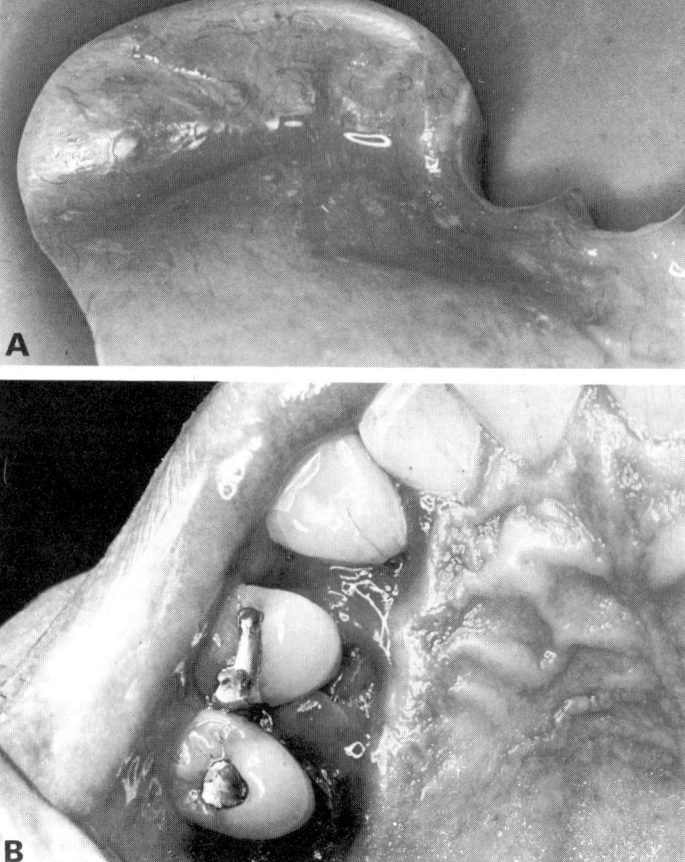

Fig. 118 (A) The close adaption of the acrylic baseplate to the teeth in a series of collets. (B) Destruction of the gingival attachments caused by this denture base.

Appendix

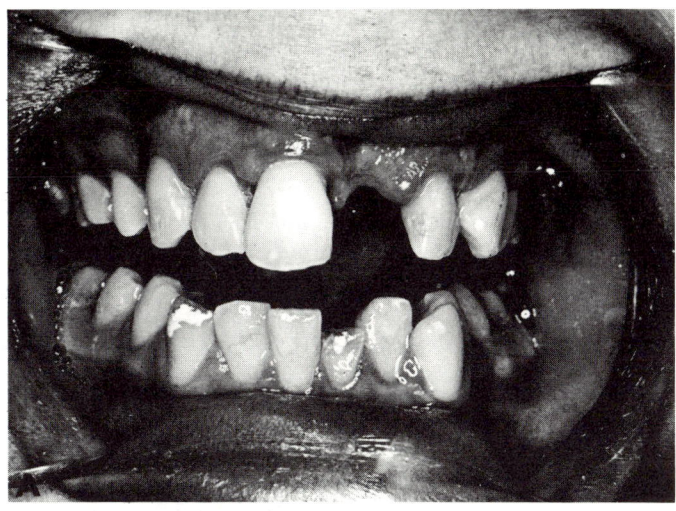

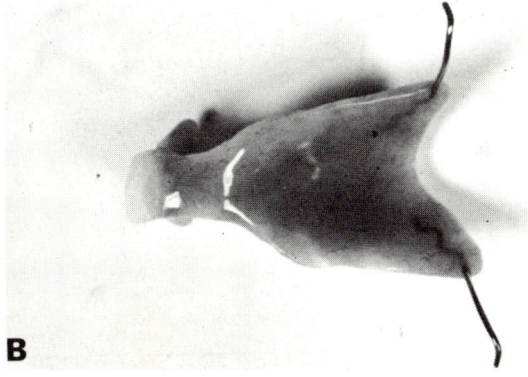

Fig. 119 (A) A mouth from which 1̲| had been lost as a result of a road traffic accident: other dental damage may also be seen. (B) The Every style denture made for this mouth.

position as undercuts are engaged. This mode of obtaining retention by movement of teeth rather than flexure of clasp arms has an obvious deleterious effect upon the periodontal health of the teeth.

Mechanical trauma is also said to cause the type of gingival damage depicted in Fig. 118. This style of colletted mucosal-borne denture, known colloquially as a 'gum stripper', moves under the influence of soft tissue displacement during chewing and, it is postulated, prises the gingival attachment from the enamel. Continued alveolar resorption beneath a mucosal-borne denture alters the relationship between collets and the gingival margin, producing a further mechanism for tissue damage.

This theory does not offer a total explanation as some mouths are encountered where a colletted denture has had no deleterious effect

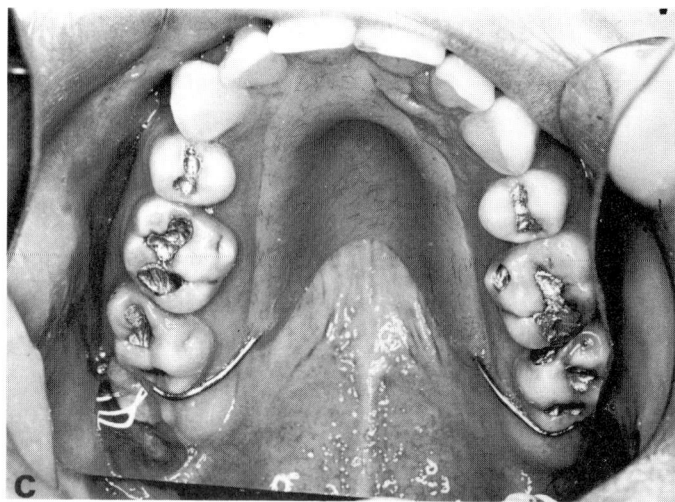

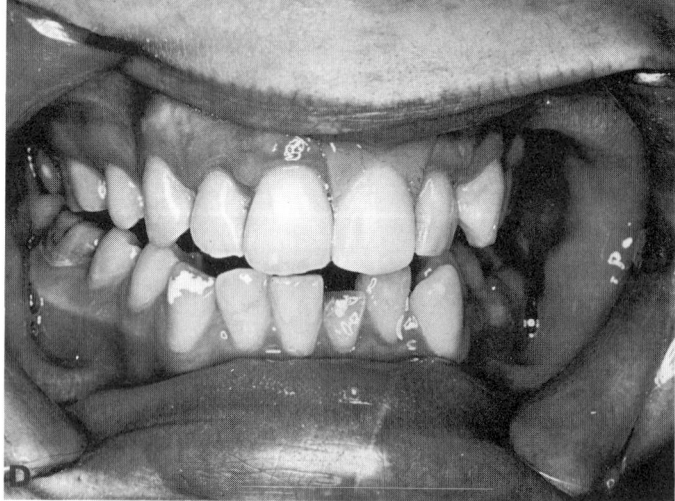

Fig. 119 (C) The denture *in situ*, showing the wrought wire components which prevent anterior displacement of the denture and the clearance of the denture base from the gingival margins. (D) Anterior view of the denture *in situ*. The presence of a flange enables tooth length to be matched accurately and prevents posterior displacement of the denture.

on the gingival tissues and yet other patients present with muco-gingival damage out of all proportion to the degree of denture displacement. Current thought suggests that the role of the collets as plaque-harbouring agents is probably as important as their potential for causing mechanical damage. Thus, where the standard of oral and denture hygiene is high, periodontal breakdown is less likely to occur.

Appendix

Principles of design

The factors to be considered when designing an acrylic partial denture are no different from those relating to the design of a metal-based denture and elaborated upon earlier in this volume. The design sequence is thus identical.

The all-acrylic partial denture is more commonly mucosal-borne, but may be tooth-borne. In the latter case, the necessary rests may be either wrought or cast; a three-armed clasp incorporating an occlusal rest is more properly cast, as a wrought rest is difficult to fit accurately to the occlusal contour. One of the problems of an acrylic base is that it is weakened by the inclusion of multiple minor connectors—a factor to be borne in mind when relating design and materials.

For the mucosally supported denture, there are two major considerations:

1 The base must be well clear of the gingival margins wherever possible. Those margins which have to be covered should be relieved, but remember that this alone is insufficient protection for the tissue. In the absence of meticulous oral hygiene, inflammation will soon occur and the gingival margins will enlarge readily to fill the relief chamber in the fit surface of the denture.

2 Maximum support must be derived from the tissues by correct extension of the denture base.

Every (1949) suggested an acrylic partial denture design for the replacement of anterior teeth which demonstrated these two principles (Fig. 119, A–D).

Features to note are:
1 Denture base at least 3 mm free of the palatal gingivae.
2 Extension of the base to the displaceable mucosa in the region of the fovea palatinae.
3 Labial flange to aid retention and brace the denture against distal movement.
4 Wrought wires to the distal margins of the posterior teeth to brace against forward movement of the denture.

Every's design incorporated the gingival protection features of the 'spoon' denture (Fig. 120), with enhanced retention and stability and was intended specifically for the replacement of anterior teeth.

Fig. 121 demonstrates how this concept may be extended to multisaddle acrylic dentures. It is just as necessary to plan the retention of an acrylic partial denture with the aid of a surveyed

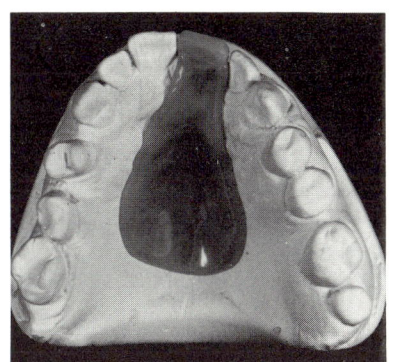

Fig. 120 The 'spoon' denture relies on adhesion for retention and is poorly braced. The advantage of the design is that palatal gingival margins are protected from trauma.

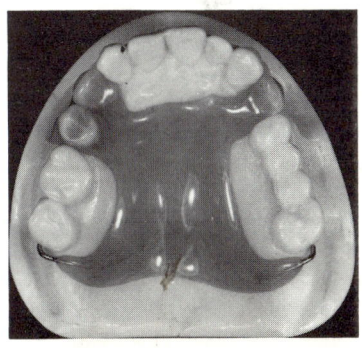

Fig. 121 A clasp-less, mucosal-borne partial denture made to a planned path of insertion. The wrought wires distally act as bracing agents. Note that the base is clear of the gingival margins wherever possible.

Partial dentures

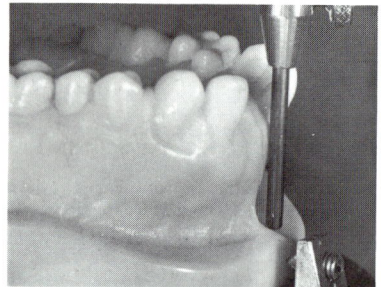

Fig. 122 This labial undercut may be engaged by a flange, if the path of insertion is correctly chosen.

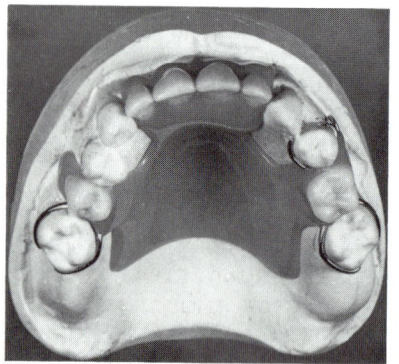

Fig. 123 The use of two-armed clasps on a mucosal-borne denture.

study cast, as it is with a metal-based denture. If, for example, the cast can be orientated on the surveyor so that a labial flange could engage the anterior alveolar undercut (Fig. 122), then some retentive quality will be conferred upon the base. In addition, the base will be braced against distal movement. When an acrylic denture is planned to a surveyed cast, unwanted undercuts may be blocked out with plaster on the processing cast. Thus, the clinician may insert the denture without the necessity of easing away excess acrylic and in the knowledge that the base will retain to an optimal extent using planned undercuts. Because of the need to block out some proximal undercuts, peripheral seal does not have a role in retaining the acrylic partial denture. A correctly extended base will not only provide optimal support, but it will also provide the maximum surface area to aid retention by adhesion.

In the case of multisaddle dentures, it is often difficult to obtain a common path of insertion which is at variance with the path of vertical displacement (see p. 26). In such an instance, the positioning of clasps is essential to the retention of the prosthesis (Fig. 123). For the mucosal-borne denture, these will be two armed occlusally-approaching or combination clasps. The clasp connectors should be embedded in the thicker acrylic of the denture saddles, as their presence creates stress in the acrylic during processing. Such stress would weaken the thinner sections of acrylic, as in the palate. The occlusal area of artificial posterior teeth carried by a mucosal-borne base should be smaller than that of the teeth they replace. The reduced resistance to food penetration by the smaller occlusal table in turn reduces the masticatory load falling upon the support tissue.

Acrylic lower partial dentures

There are a number of problems in achieving an effective design of acrylic lower partial dentures. The major difficulty is one of gaining adequate support, especially where the denture is mucosal-borne. In the latter instance it is necessary to extend the base in the edentulous regions as one would for a complete denture. The load is spread as widely as possible by extending the base to the external oblique ridges and by covering the buccal shelves. Posteriorly, the extension should cover at least one-third of the retromolar pads. Failure to observe these precautions will cause excessive load to be transmitted to the alveolar bone, producing accelerated resorption.

Where there are posterior saddles with anterior standing teeth, a

Appendix

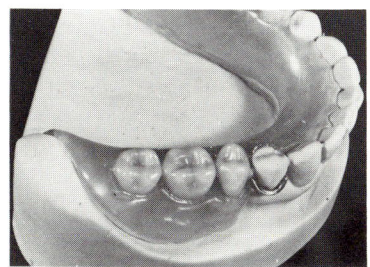

Fig. 124 There are hazards to gingival health in this style of mucosal-borne lower partial denture.

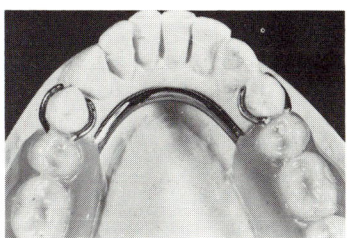

Fig. 125 The lingual bar leaves the gingival margins uncovered, but there must be generous spacing between the inferior aspect of the bar and the floor of the mouth. In the absence of rests on the abutment teeth, the bar may sink and traumatise the lingual mucosa.

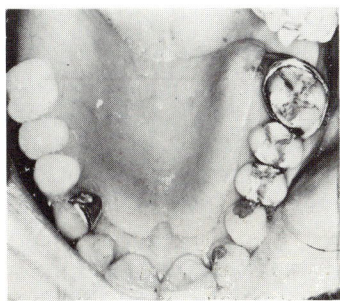

Fig. 126 The clasp to |6 and the bracing arm to 3| are cast elements which have been incorporated ...as acrylic design.

commonly encountered major connector is a thickened lingual plate (Fig. 124). This is closely adapted to the lingual aspect of the lower anterior teeth and the gingival margins. When the mucosal-borne denture is subjected to load and there is movement of the base due to mucosal displacement, a shearing force is applied to the natural teeth and their gingival margins. Tissue morbidity may be reduced by replacing the acrylic connector with a wrought lingual bar where appropriate (Fig. 125). However, there must be generous spacing inferior to the bar and tooth support must be provided so that it does not press into the floor of the mouth as the patient chews.

The choice of acrylic as the denture base material places further constraints on the effective design of a lower partial denture. Indirect retention, when required, is difficult to achieve without a bulky acrylic lingual plate. When occlusal rests are included in the design to confer tooth support, an adequate thickness of acrylic must surround the connectors so that the denture base is not weakened too much. This necessity for increasing the bulk of the prosthesis so that it may have adequate strength results in a greater awareness of the denture by the patient.

A means of incorporating retaining and supporting elements into an acrylic-based denture without complicating the design is to cast these components with their connectors in cobalt-chrome alloy. Wax patterns may be prepared on the stone master cast, sprued and lifted off gently to be attached to the sprue former of a major casting which is about to be invested in the laboratory. Fig. 126 illustrates how such a cast retainer and connector incorporated into an upper, mucosal-borne acrylic partial denture enables palatal gingival margins to remain unencumbered by the denture base.

Special notes on specific forms of partial denture design

TWO-PART DENTURES

The small bounded edentulous space may create problems for the patient from the point of view of appearance or eating. Unilateral dentures ('side plates') are unsatisfactory prostheses as retention is frequently inadequate and the absence of cross-arch bracing renders them unstable. Due to their small size, they might be swallowed or inhaled if accidentally dislodged. Bridge work might be considered as the treatment of choice in these circumstances unless there are contraindications. These might include the youth of the patient where the pulp chamber would be large, the undesirability of removing quantities of healthy tissue in the preparation of abutment teeth or the unfavourable orientation of an abutment tooth. The two-part denture is a useful prosthesis to meet this situation. There are various forms but the principle is the same for all. A requirement which has to be met is the presence of adequate approximal undercuts and, in the case of an anterior denture, a labial alveolar undercut. The two components of the denture are designed for insertion along differing paths so that the maximum amount of tissue undercut is engaged. When the components are locked together, the prosthesis is rigidly retained.

Locking mechanisms

Two systems are in use, the bolt and friction locking devices. The former was the first system to be used, but has the disadvantage that it loosens in service due to wear and is not readily adjustable (Fig. 127). The bolt is positioned in the acrylic flange of part 'b' of the denture and locks into a hole provided in the metal casting of part 'a'. The bolt is so designed that it cannot be withdrawn unless the handle is lifted—the components of the denture are therefore not liable to fall apart in use.

The friction locking devices may be either of a 'split pin' type, individually prepared for the denture, or a precision attachment (e.g. the Conod) (Figs. 128, 129) soldered to the metal base of part 'a'. The pin, or attachment, is paralleled to the path of insertion of part 'b' and is accepted by a sleeve in that part. The patient may be provided

Special notes on specific forms of partial denture design 105

with a key to assist with the removal of part 'b': the pegs on the key fit into slots positioned on the labial flange above the smile line.

Anterior tooth replacement

The treatment illustrated in Fig. 127, A–E demonstrates features of a two-part design based on the locking bolt system. The metal plate

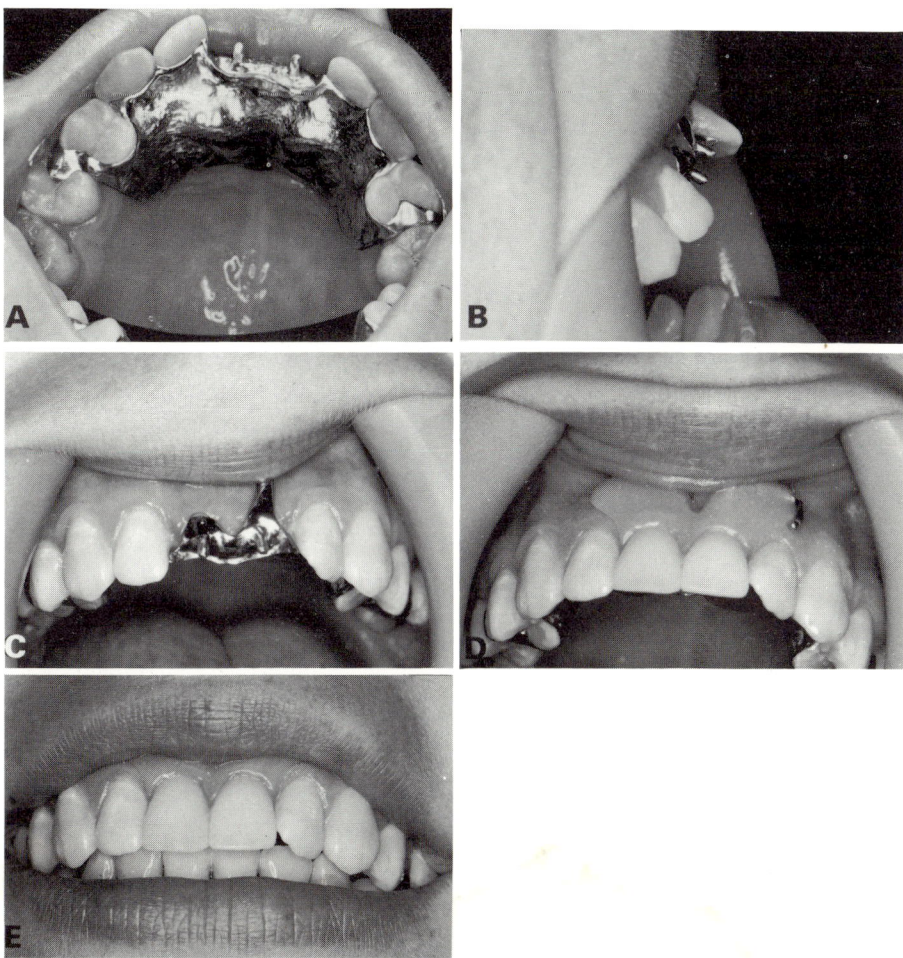

Fig. 127 (A) Part 'a' of a locking bolt two-part denture *in situ*. (B) The orientation of the guide posts. (C) The spur carrying a hole for the locking bolt. (D) Part 'b' *in situ* with the bolt locked. (E) The appearance of the denture.

Partial dentures

(part 'a') is tooth-borne and carries discrete interstitial clasps between the premolar teeth of each side. These clasps serve to retain the denture posteriorly and also aid in bracing the denture against anteroposterior displacement.

The two posts in the region of the replacement teeth promote internal rigidity of the assembled posthesis: as they have the additional function of aiding the location of the second part of the denture (part 'b'), their orientation is paralleled to its path of insertion (B). The metal base also carries a spur which extends into the labial sulcus and which carries the hole for the locking bolt and its extremity (C). Part 'b' carries the artificial teeth (sleeved internally to accept the posts of part 'a') and the labial flange, into which is incorporated the locking bolt (D). The bolt handle is prepared to the distal aspect of the labial flange above the smile line, and should not detract from the appearance of the prosthesis (E). The advantage of using posts to brace the internal structure of the prosthesis is that transmitted light may still pass through the replacement teeth, permitting a faithful colour match. The components of single-tooth dentures are more difficult to brace mutually. Part 'a' is thus designed with a post and palatal flange aligned to the path of insertion of part 'b' to achieve this end. Fig. 128 illustrates such a situation, in this instance with a split-pin locking device. The palatal flange should not extend to the incisal edge of the replacement tooth, as translucency will be lost. Unless care is taken, the body colour of the tooth will also be darkened by the necessary presence of the metal flange. The use of the Conod attachment as a friction locking device is shown in Fig. 129, A. The additional post enhances the rigidity of the structures. The two perforations high on the labial flange accept the key which facilitates separation of the components on removal of the denture (Fig. 129, B).

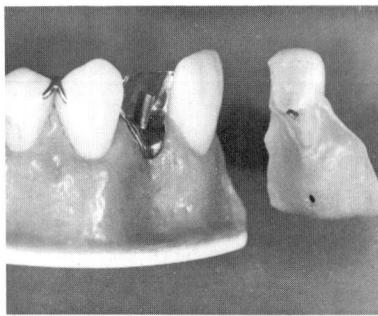

Fig. 128 A split-pin locking device for an anterior two-part denture.

Special notes on specific forms of partial denture design 107

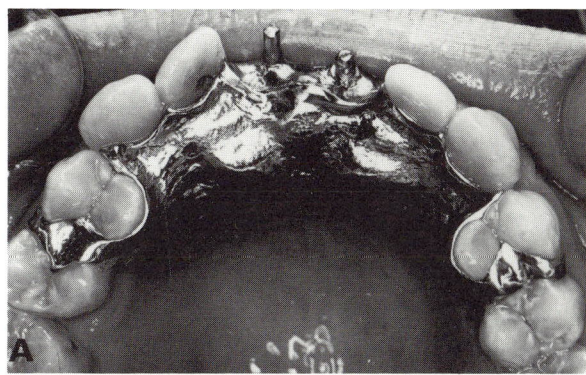

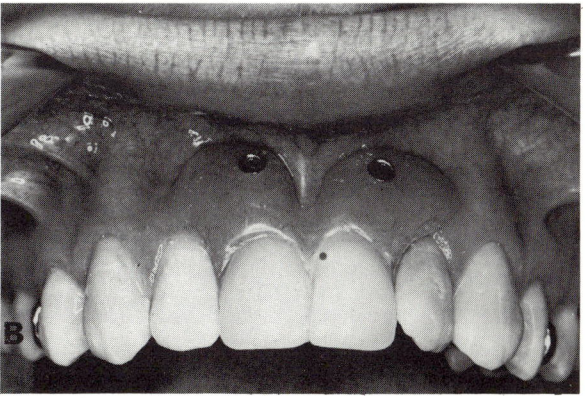

Fig. 129 (A) A Conod attachment (right) used as a locking device. (B) Perforations in the flange of part 'b' to aid its removal.

Posterior tooth replacement

An edentulous space suited to this form of restoration would be bounded by abutment teeth with a good height of clinical crown and well marked approximal undercuts (Fig. 130). Part 'a' of the denture is inserted along an inferoposterior path of insertion to engage the mesial undercut of the distal abutment (Fig. 131, A). This component carries an anterior strut which serves both as a minor connector for the occlusal rest and also to brace the denture against posterior movement. The hole for the locking bolt to engage is prepared in the distal facet of this component. The facet is paralleled to the distal shape of the medial abutment to act as a guide plane for the insertion of part 'b'. This second part carries the replacement teeth, buccal flange bearing the locking bolt, occlusal rests to the distal aspects of both abutment teeth and additional bracing arms (Fig. 131, B). The form of these arms may vary according to the

Partial dentures

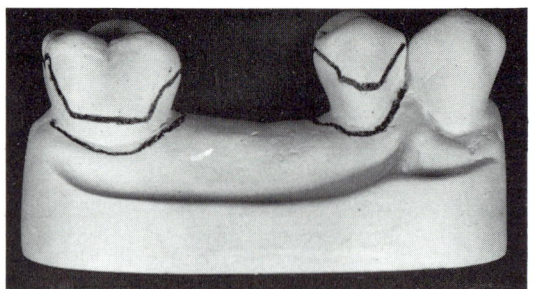

Fig. 130 A two-part prosthesis would be a suitable restoration for this edentulous space.

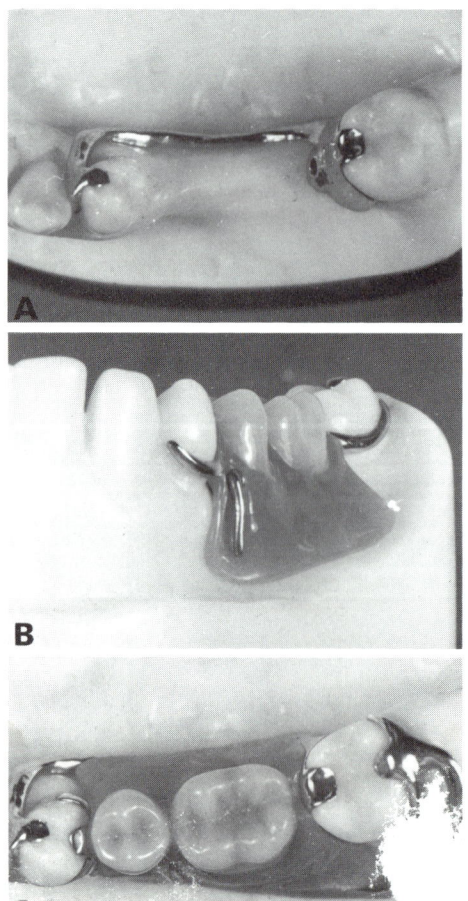

Fig. 131 (A) The positioning of part 'a' of a posterior two-part denture. (B) Part 'b' locked in position. (C) Occlusal view showing an alternative means of planning retention and buccolingual bracing.

Special notes on specific forms of partial denture design

survey marking on the abutment teeth: an occlusal view of an assembled denture (Fig. 131, C) shows an alternative configuration.

HINGED FLANGE DENTURES

These are a variation of the two-part design and have similar indications for use. The teeth and buccal flange are mounted on a hinge axis. The denture is inserted 'open' (Fig. 132, A), allowing the metal base to be inserted along its most favourable path. For example for an anterior saddle this path may be horizontal, permitting approximal undercuts of the abutment teeth to be engaged. Closure of the flange enables the labial alveolar undercut to be engaged and the components are locked in the 'closed' position by a bolt (Fig. 132, B). Difficulty may be encountered with this design when anterior teeth are spaced, or require to be set to a pronounced curve of the arch. In such instances, a single, long hinge is inappropriate and the teeth are hinged to paralleled posts set into their palatal aspect (Fig. 133).

As with two-part dentures, the hinge flange prosthesis designed for posterior saddles must be well supported by the abutment teeth and adequately braced. With buccal clasp arms attached to the hinged flange (Fig. 134, A), it is possible to engage deep undercuts which would not be accessible to conventional clasps (Fig. 134, B). Although the principle of the posterior hinge flange denture may be appreciated readily, its production demands a technical exactness. The positioning of the hinge axis, for example, must be precise if the teeth are not to restrict the opening of the denture by contact of the lingual cusps against the metal lingual flange on 'opening' the denture. The hinged flange or two-part systems need not be

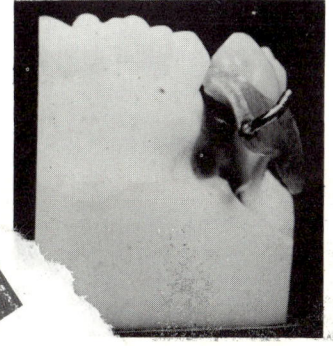 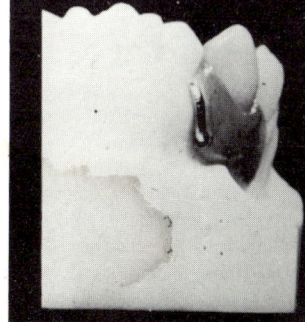

Fig. 132 (A) The insertion of a hinged flange denture. (B) The flange 'closed' with the locking bolt in place.

Partial dentures

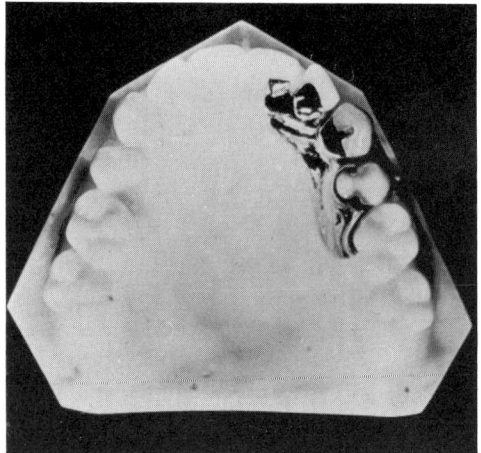

Fig. 133 The left canine tooth is individually hinged to the denture about the post set into its palatal aspect. This has enabled the denture to be made with interproximal spacing of the replacement tooth.

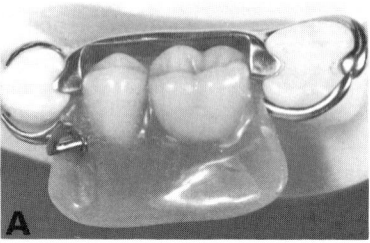

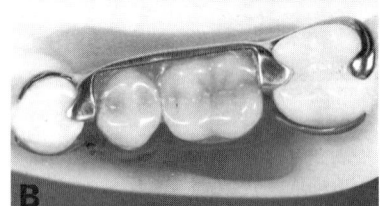

Fig. 134 (A) A hinged flanged posterior denture 'open' for insertion. The axis of the hinge is parallel with the residual ridge crest, whilst the locking bolt handle is elevated in the 'unlocked' position. (B) The denture 'closed'.

confined in their application to small dentures for single saddles. They are convenient to use for the replacement of anterior teeth in multi-saddle dentures when they confer excellent retention without the use of prominent clasps (Fig. 135).

THE SWINGLOCK DENTURE

This type of appliance which was introduced by Simmons (1963) is particularly useful when the only undercut areas are near to the

Special notes on specific forms of partial denture design

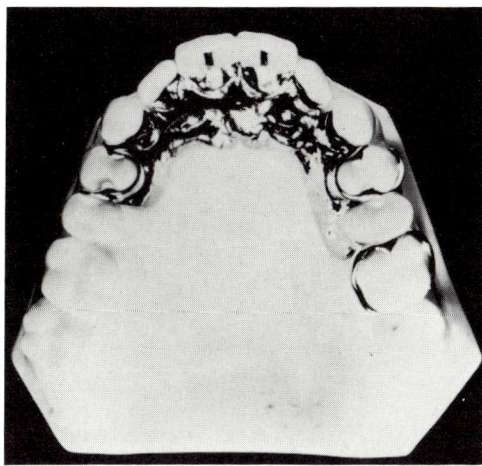

Fig. 135 A hinged anterior flange on a denture which also replaces an upper premolar and carries conventional clasps.

gingival margins on the labial aspect of remaining anterior teeth (Fig. 136, A, B). It provides splinting for the teeth and by the use of an acrylic labial veneer may be used following mucogingival surgery when the design of the denture masks any unsightly lengthening of the natural clinical crowns (Fig. 137, A, B). It may be used in association with overdentures when copings are prepared on the endodontically treated roots as shown in Fig. 138, A–C. Bolender and Becker (1981) and Stewart *et al.* (1983) suggest the following indications for the Swinglock technique:

1 Inadequate bone support for key abutment teeth.

2 Missing key abutments, e.g. a missing canine forces the use of a lateral incisor as an abutment.

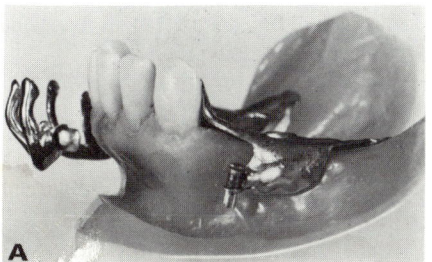 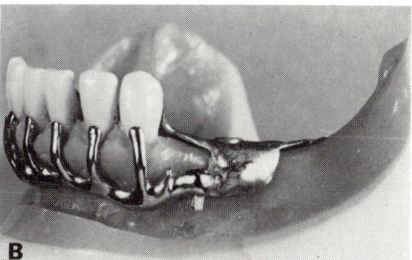

Fig. 136 (A) The lingual framework has been designed about a path of insertion parallel to the distal surface of the distal abutment. (B) The labial segment rotates horizontally with its bar in a tissue undercut and the projecting 'T' bars making contact with the teeth below the survey line. This type of design may be employed even when the canine is missing.

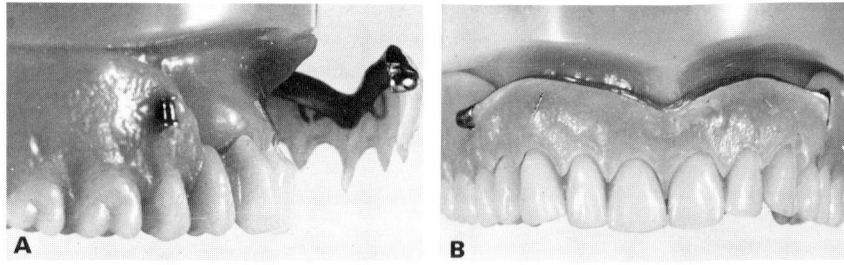

Fig. 137 (A and B) Recession of the gingival tissue has left unsightly spaces between the upper anterior teeth. The bar carries acrylic gumwork which restores a pleasing appearance.

3   The presence of mobile teeth which may or may not be abutment teeth.
4   Inadequate undercuts on potential abutment teeth adjacent to edentulous areas.
5   Where splinting is required and the economic resources of the patient prohibit fixed splinting.
6   There are too few remaining natural teeth for a conventionally designed removable partial denture.
7   Retention and stabilisation for maxillofacial prosthesis.

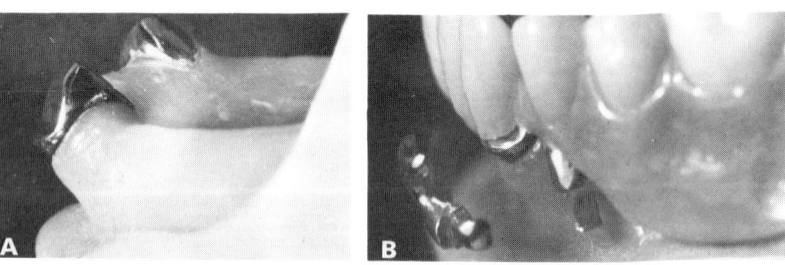

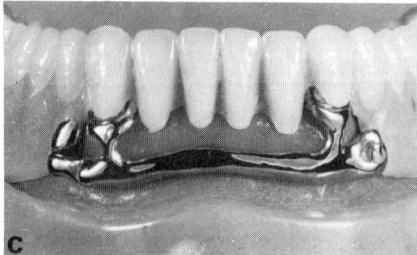

Fig. 138 (A and C) Two endodontically treated lower canines support copings which provide a guide plane for the lingual segment and an undercut which is engaged by the labial component.

Special notes on specific forms of partial denture design

8 Positions of remaining teeth are not favourable for a conventional design, e.g. malposed teeth.

9 As a provisional splint during periodontal therapy when fixed splinting is being considered.

The Swinglock denture framework is fitted with a hinged labial flange which is closely adapted to the cervical aspects of the remaining anterior teeth. With the hinge open, the denture is inserted from the occlusal direction. With the denture base seated, the hinged flange is rotated horizontally to engage the tooth undercuts, being maintained in this position by a snap lock at its extremity. To ensure that the denture cannot move towards the gingival tissues, it is essential that adequate tooth support is provided. It should be borne in mind that the path of insertion of the labio-gingival element is on an arc determined by the hinge. This may necessitate some easing of the fitting surface to allow it to enter undercuts without stressing the teeth. Because this type of denture splints the teeth so firmly it is important that any distal extension saddle is well supported and does not displace excessively during chewing. The fluid wax impression technique described in Clinical stage 3A should be adopted to ensure that no stress is transmitted to the remaining natural teeth.

DISJUNCT DENTURES

Disjunct dentures are a useful means of overcoming support problems in the partially edentulous mouth, especially when the remaining teeth are of poor periodontal prognosis. The denture is of two components, a tooth-borne retaining splint and a mucosal-borne base. The former is recessed into the latter, but the parts are not locked together and the mucosal-borne denture base can move as a result of mucosal displacement independently of the retaining splint. A brief description of the production of a disjunct denture for a bilateral distal extension saddle situation in the upper jaw will illustrate features of the design.

The usual clinical procedures are followed through the primary and secondary impressions, jaw relations and trial insertion stages: a temporary self-cure resin or shellac base may be used for the latter two. A new wax base of two sheets of 0·7 mm high fusing sheet wax (e.g. Wipla blue) is laid down on the duplicate cast. The sheets are adapted individually, the first being trimmed 3 mm clear of the gingival margins of the standing teeth (Fig. 139).

The form into which the retaining splint will be inlaid is cut from the second thickness of wax, leaving a 3 mm shelf anteriorly. The

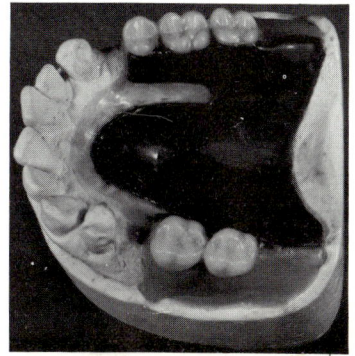

Fig. 139 The wax pattern for the base is laid down in two thicknesses of 0·7 mm sheetwax. The form of the retaining splint is cut from the second thickness of wax and the base is 3 mm clear of all gingival margins.

Partial dentures

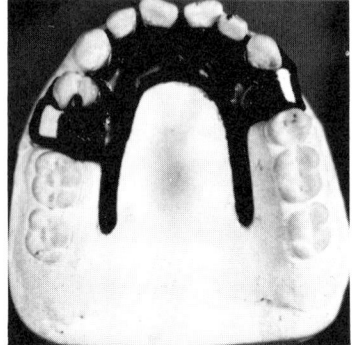

Fig. 140 An investment cast is made from the stage illustrated in Fig.128. The wax pattern of the retaining splint is laid down on the investment cast.

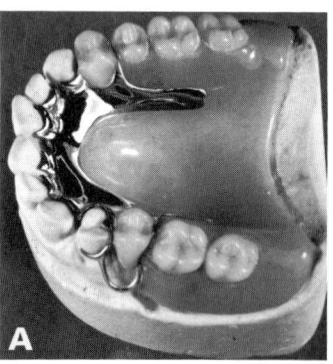

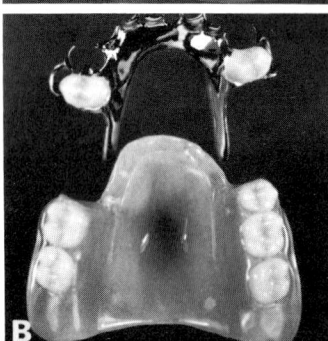

Fig. 141 (A) The disjunct denture assembled on the master cast. (B) The disassembled components of the disjunct dentures.

borders of the cut-away portion should be prepared with a 5° flare and the splint must be designed so that the denture base cannot be displaced distally beneath it. The cast is then returned to the articulator and the posterior teeth reset on the new wax base: two replacement teeth approximal to the abutment teeth are not reset (Fig. 139).

The waxed-up denture is then sealed to the cast and duplicated in investment medium. The wax pattern for the retaining splint may then be laid on the investment cast overlaying the anterior shelf of the mucosal-borne component. Clasp design is dictated by tooth contour: should this be unfavourable, then inlays may be fitted for ball and dimple bar clasps. The splint is tooth-borne through the agency of occlusal and cingulum rests. Provision should be made for the attachment of the two replacement teeth which are to be carried by this component (Fig. 140). After waxing up, the splint is cast in cobalt-chromium alloy and finished in the usual way. The completed splint is fitted to the master cast, overlaying the waxed-up denture base, which is then processed in acrylic around the splint. The two remaining teeth, cantilevered from the tooth-borne component of the denture, are set up and processed to the splint with self-cure resin: provided the recessing for the retaining splint was not undercut in the wax pattern, the metal should come away from the acrylic base without difficulty (Fig. 141).

The following points are of significance:

1 The mucosal-borne base can move as support tissue is displaced without traumatising gingival margins.

2 The gingival margins are covered by the tooth-borne component of the denture. There is no danger of the gingival attachment being stripped from the teeth and there are no relieved areas into which the gingival tissue may proliferate.

3 The tooth-borne component may be used to splint the anterior teeth, either by parallel pins which fit into prepared sleeves in the cingulae or through the agency of incisal rests (unsightly).

4 Apart from any splinting function, the tooth-borne component is an excellent retainer for the denture. It is retained in position by conventional clasps but the posterior extension arms, inlaid into the acrylic base, prevent the mucosal component from rotating around an axis passing through the abutment teeth. This problem is one which is frequently difficult to solve (without gingival damage) in conventional mucosal and tooth-borne and mucosal-borne designs.

References and further reading

ACADEMY OF DENTURE PROSTHETICS (1963) Principles, concepts and practices in Prosthodontics—Progress Report III. *Journal of Prosthetic Dentistry*, **13**, 283–294.

APPLEGATE C.C. (1959) Completing the master cast. In *Essentials of Removable Partial Prostheses*, 2nd edn, pp. 299–312, Saunders, Philadelphia.

ATKINSON H.F. (1953) Partial denture problems. Designing about a path of withdrawal. *Australian Journal of Dentistry*, **57**, 187–190.

BOLENDER, C.L. & BECKER, C.M. (1981) Swinglock removable partial dentures, where and when? *Journal of Prosthetic Dentistry*, **45**, 1.

BRILL, N., TRYDE, G., STOLTZE, K. & EL GHAMRANY, E.A. (1977) Ecological changes in the oral cavity caused by removable partial dentures. *Journal of Prosthetic Dentistry*, **38**, 138–148.

CARLSSON G.E., HEDEGÅRD B. & KOIVUMAA K.K. (1960) Studies in partial dental prosthesis I. An investigation of dentogingivally supported partial dentures. *Suomen Hammaslääkäriseuran Toimituksia*, **56**, 248–306.

CARLSSON G.E., HEDEGÅRD B. & KOIVUMAA K.K. (1961) Studies in partial dental prosthesis II. An investigation of mandibular partial dentures with double extension saddles. *Acta Odontologica Scandinavica*, **19**, 215–237.

CARLSSON G.E., HEDEGÅRD B. & KOIVUMAA K.K. (1962) Studies in partial dental prosthesis III. A longitudinal study of mandibular partial dentures with double extension saddles. *Acta Odontologica Scandinavica*, **20**, 95–119.

CECCONI B.T. (1974) Effect of rest design on transmission of forces to abutment teeth. *Journal of Prosthetic Dentistry*, **32**, 141–151.

COSTA E. (1970) A simplified system for identifying partially edentulous dental arches. *Journal of Prosthetic Dentistry*, **32**, 639–645.

COY R.E. & ARNOLD P.D. (1974) Survey and design of diagnostic casts for removable partial dentures. *Journal of Prosthetic Dentistry*, **32**, 103–106.

CUMMER, W.E. (1920) Possible combinations of teeth present and missing in partial restorations. *Oral Health*, **10**, 421–430.

EVERY R.G. (1949) The elimination of destructive forces in replacing teeth with partial dentures. *New Zealand Dental Journal*, **45**, 207–214.

GEISSLER P.R. & WATT D.M. (1965) Disjunct dentures for patients with teeth of poor prognosis. *Dental Practitioner*, **15**, 421–423.

HENDERSON D. (1966) Writing work authorizations for removable partial dentures. *Journal of Prosthetic Dentistry*, **16**, 696–707.

HENDERSON D. & STEFFEL V.L. (eds.) (1970) *McCracken's Removable Partial Prosthodontics*, 4th edn, Mosby, St Louis.

HOWE G.L. (1971) Surgical aids to denture construction. In *Minor Oral Surgery* 2nd edn, pp. 208–233, Wright, Bristol.

KENNEDY E.J. (1928) Classification of partially edentulous arches. In *Partial Denture Construction*, pp. 3–8, Dental Items of Interest, Brooklyn N.Y.

KRATOCHVIL P.J. (1963) Influence of occlusal rest position and clasp design on movement of abutment teeth. *Journal of Prosthetic Dentistry*, **13**, 114–124.

LEE J.H. (1963) Sectional partial metal dentures incorporating an internal locking bolt. *Journal of Prosthetic Dentistry*, **13**, 1067–1075.

L'ESTRANGE P.R. & WARNER E. (1969) Sectional dentures: a simplified method of attachment. *Dental Practitioner*, **19**, 379–381.

L'ESTRANGE P.R. & WARNER E. (1969) Sectional dentures: aids to removal and adjustment. *Dental Practitioner*, **20**, 135–138.

MCCRACKEN W.L. (1956) Mouth preparation for partial dentures. *Journal of Prosthetic Dentistry*, **6**, 38–52.

MCCRORIE, J.W. (1982) Corrective impression waxes. *British Dental Journal*, **152**, 95–96.

NAIRN R.I. (1966) The problem of free-end denture bases. *Journal of Prosthetic Dentistry*, **16**, 522–532.

NEILL D.J. (1958) The problem of the lower free-end removable partial denture. *Journal of Prosthetic Dentistry*, **8**, 623–634.

RANTANEN, T., SIIRILA, H.S. & LEHRILA, P. (1980) Effect of instruction and motivation on dental knowledge and behaviour among wearers of partial dentures. *Acta Odontologica Scandinavica*, **38**, 9–15.

ROACH F.E. (1930) Principles and essentials of bar clasp partial dentures. *Journal of the American Dental Association*, **17**, 124–138.

RUDD K.D. & O'LEARY T.J. (1966) Stabilising periodontally weakened teeth by using guide plane removable partial dentures. *Journal of Prosthetic Dentistry*, **16**, 721–727.

SIMMONS, J.J. (1963) Swinglock stabilization and retention. *Texas Dental Journal*, **81**, 10–17.

SKINNER C.N. (1959) A classification of removable partial dentures based upon principles of anatomy and physiology. *Journal of Prosthetic Dentistry*, **9**, 240–384.

STEWART, K., RUDD, K.D. & KUEBKER, W.A. (1983) *Clinical Removable Partial Prosthodontics*, C.V. Mosby, St. Louis, pp. 588–624.

STIPHO, M.D.K., MURPHY, W.M. & ADAMS, D. (1978) Effect of oral prostheses on plaque accumulation. *British Dental Journal*, **145**, 47–50.

WALTER J.D. (1971) An assessment of alginate materials. *Dental Practitioner*, **21**, 377–384.

WARNER, E.P. & L'ESTRANGE, P.R. (1978) *Sectional Dentures*, Wright, Bristol.

WATT D.M., MACGREGOR A.R., GEDDES M., COCKBURN A. & BOYD J.L. (1958) A preliminary investigation of the support of partial dentures and its relationship to vertical loads. *Dental Practitioner*, **9**, 1–15.

ZARB, G.A. & MACKAY, H.F. (1980) The biologic price of prosthodontic intervention. *Australian Dental Journal*, **25**, 63–68.

Index

Number prefixed by 'f' indicates figure

Acrylic base
  construction procedure 97
  design 98, 101
  lower dentures 102
  mucosal borne 99, 101
Adams crib clasps 42, f50
Adjustments to dentures 94–5
  instruments and materials 92
Alginate impression(s)
  casting 23–4
  material 9, 11, 12
  procedure 9–15
Alveolar process, resorption 96
Amphotericin B in denture related stomatitis 51
Anaemia, oral signs 7, 8
Anterior tooth replacement
  by two part denture 105–7
  denture design for 39, 40
  path of insertion for 26
  selection of teeth 85
Anticoagulants and dental treatment 5
Applegate fluid wax technique 80–3
Articulator, mounting casts f31, 29

Bar clasps *see* Clasps, bar
Bar connectors *see* Connectors, bar
Bleeding, excessive, and dental treatment 5
Bracing, cross arch 39

Candidal infection, oral 8, f58
Canine teeth, support potential 32–3
Caries 6, 91
  inspection for 6, 95
Cast, master
  altering with fluid wax impression 83
  duplicating in investment 59
  hydrocol duplicate of 62
  outlining design on 59
  preparation of 57 *et seq.*

Cast, master (*cont.*)
  relieving 60
  surveying 57–9
Cast framework
  casting 67
  distal extension saddle 75–8
  finishing 68
  investing 66
  'stress breaking' 33, 75–6, 78
  trial insertion 72, 74–5
  wax pattern 69
Cast, study
  mounting on articulator 29
  occlusal analysis 17
  occlusional rims on 24–5
  pouring 23
  surveying 25–9
Casting
  impressions 23–4
  metal framework 66–8
Centric occlusion 16, 18–19
  registering 18–19
Check record 95
Cingulum rest seat 54
Clasps
  Adams 42, f50
  bar 41–2
  checking 95
  circumferential 39–41
    back action 40
    C form f41, 40
    encircling 41
    extended arm 40
    recurved 40
    reverse back action 40
  cobalt chromium material for, 35
  combination 42, f48
  'continuous' 37
  crib 42, f50
  design 39, 43–4
  embrasure 42–3
  gingivally approaching 41–2, 75
  occlusally approaching *see* circumferential

Clasps (*cont.*)
  positioning 35–7
  retention provided by 34–7
  ring (encircling) *see* circumferential
  Roach 41–2
  on two-part dentures 106
  undercut gauge 58
  wrought gold 35
Classification of edentulous spaces 30, f32
Cobalt–chromium alloys
  denture bases 59
Collet f118, 98
  mechanical damage associated with 99
  plaque-harbouring agents 100
Connectors
  bar 44–5, 46
  continuous f38
  design 44–5
  labial bar 46, f54
  plate 44, 46–7
Conod attachment 104, 106
Crib clasps *see* Clasps, crib
Cross-arch bracing 39
Crowns, artificial, to assist retention 36

Denture
  casting and finishing framework 66–9
  damage to 95
  handling 92
  lining with tissue conditioner 51
  stomatitis 50, 51
Diabetes and dental treatment 5
Diet 93
Disclosing tablets 92
Disjunct dentures 113–14
Displacement, resistance to 34–7
  direct retainers 34–7
  indirect retainers 37, f39

117

Index

Drugs and dental treatment 5
Dry mouth 6

Edentulous spaces, classification 30, f32
Elasticity, modulus of 35
Electrobrightening of metal framework 69–71
Encircling clasps *see* Clasps, circumferential
Epilepsy and design of denture 5
Every style denture f119, 101
Examination
  extraoral 6
  intraoral 6–8

Facebow
  assembly f17
  record 16
Ferrous gluconate in iron deficiency treatment 51
Finishing and polishing cast framework 68–71
Fitting completed dentures 90–91
Fluid wax technique 80–2
  Applegate 78, 80–2
  McCrorie's recipe 81
Food
  and partial dentures 93
  stagnation zones 30, 54, f101
Fremitus 7

Gingiva, damage to f118, 99
  pressure on 95
Gingivally approaching clasps *see* Clasps, gingivally approaching
Gold, wrought, as clasp material 35
Guide planes 25–6, 35, 36, 37

Handling dentures 92
Heart disease and dental treatment 5
Hinged flange dentures 109–11
History, patient's
  dental 6
  medical 5–6
Hydrocal duplicate of master cast 62
Hygiene, denture and oral 91–2, 100

Impression tray, selection 9, 10
Impressions
  alginate, casting of 23–4
  alginate impression procedure 9–15
  boxing prior to casting 57
  primary 8–15
    lower 14–16
    upper 9–14
  wax for distal extension saddle 81–2
  working, after mouth preparation 56
Insertion
  path of 33–4
  trial 87
  setting teeth for trial 86
Investing wax pattern 66
Investment cast, preparing 59–62
Investment, liquid 66
Iron deficiency, anaemia 51

Jaw relationships 16–18, 84–6
  selection of teeth 85
  see also Retruded contact position

Kennedy
  bar 37
  classification of edentulous spaces 30, f32

Locking mechanisms *see* two-part dentures
Lower incisor abutment tooth as support 33

Mandibular closure 17
Masticatory load and partial denture design 32–3
Medical history 5–6
Metal framework, investing and casting 66–8
  finishing for mouth insertion 68–71
Modulus of elasticity of clasps 35
Molar teeth as support 32
Mould, agar gel 61, f80–82

Mouth
  antibiotic therapy 6
  clinical examination 6–8
  preparation for partial dentures 49–52
  specific preparation 53–6
  trial insertion of cast framework in 72–5
Mucoperiosteum
  clinical examination 7
  denture adjustment for damage to 94–5
  displaced impression of 80
  masticatory load on 32–3
  support for denture 32–3, 95
Mucosal supported acrylic dentures 101–3
  deleterious effects 97
  multisaddle dentures 101
Muscle, mylohyoid 80

Nystatin in denture-related stomatitis 51

Occlusal analysis 16–18
  preparation of table 53–4
Occlusal rests 54
Occlusal wafer 18, 19, 29, 90, 95
Occlusion
  adjustment for errors 95
  modification of form 54
  registering centric 18, 20
  rims 19, 20–2
Oral hygiene 8, 51
  after denture fitting 91–2

Panelipse radiographs 7–8
Paste, for occlusal record 19
Path of insertion *see* Insertion
Periapical radiographs *see* Radiographs
Periodontal disease 91
  inspection for 7, 95
Peridontal therapy 8, 52
Plaque retention 7, 76, 78, 92
Plate connectors *see* Connectors, plate
Processing the denture 88
Provisional treatment plan 8

Index

Radiographs
  bite-wing 8
  panelipse 7–8
  periapical 8
Resistance to displacement 34–7
Resistance to horizontal plane
    movement 37, 39
Rest seats, preparation 54
  positioning 33
Retainers
  direct 34–7, *see also* Clasps
  indirect 37
  undercut gauge to determine
    position 58
Retention 34–7
  of acrylic dentures 101–2
Retruded contact position 16–8
  registering 20–2
Rheumatic fever and dental
    treatment 5
Ring clasp 41
Roach clasps 39, 41

Saddle 30–3
  anterior bounded 30, f30, f32
  areas, outline and support 27–31
  distal extension 30, f32, 75–8, 80
    acrylic tray addition 78–9
    fluid wax impression
      technique 80–3
    hinged f104
    modifying by wax impression 83
    pressure on mucoperiosteum 75
    'stress breaking' 75
    technique for recording
      impression, distal
      extension 80–2
  mucosa support for 32, 101
  tooth support for 32–3
  tooth and mucosal support for 33

Saddle (*cont.*)
  unilateral bounded 30, f32
Silica
  gel 60–1, 62
  particles 61
Sinus, in mucosa 7
Split pin locking device 104, 106
Spoon dentures, retention of 99
Spruing 64–5
  from above 65
  through model base 65
Steroids, and dental treatment 5
Stomatitis, denture 7, 50–1
  management 51–2
Stone, dental 23
Study casts
  mounting 24, f27, 29
  surveying 24–9
'Stress breaking' 75–8
Support
  mucosal 32, 101
  tooth 32–3
  tooth and mucosal 33
Surveying procedure 24–9
Surveying master casts 57–8
Surveyor 26–7
Swinglock dentures 110–13

Teeth *see* Tooth
Tissue
  assessment 7
  conditioner 51
  surgical preparation 53–4
Tongue, examination 7
Tooth
  anterior replacement by two-part
    denture 105–7
  assessment 2, 7
  form modification 54
  posterior replacement by two-part
    denture 107–9

Tooth (*cont.*)
  preparation for partial
    dentures 49–54
  selection of replacement 85
  selection to provide support for
    dentures 32, 33
Toothpaste, abrasive effect on acrylic
    resin 91
Trays, construction 47–8
Treatment planning 8, 49
Two-part dentures 104–9
  anterior tooth replacement 105–7
  disjunct 113–14
  locking mechanisms for 104, f129,
    131, 134
  posterior tooth replacement 107–9

Undercut gauge 58
Use, instructions for, of dentures 92–3

Vitamin deficiency, oral signs 7

Wax
  blocking undercut areas with 59
  boxing impressions with 57
  disclosing 72, f100, 95
  fluid, technique for impression of
    distal extension saddle
    area f105, 80–3, f111
  investing pattern 66
  McCrorie's recipe 81
  occlusal wafer, 18, 90 *see also*
    Occlusal wafer
  pattern preparation 62–4

Young's modulus of elasticity 35